ABC OF
SPINAL CORD INJURY

ABC OF
SPINAL CORD INJURY

Fourth edition

Edited by

DAVID GRUNDY

*Honorary Consultant in Spinal Injuries,
The Duke of Cornwall
Spinal Treatment Centre,
Salisbury District Hospital, UK*

ANDREW SWAIN

*Clinical Director, Emergency Department,
MidCentral Health, Palmerston Hospital North,
New Zealand*

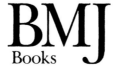

© BMJ Books 2002
BMJ Books is an imprint of the BMJ Publishing Group

BMJ Publishing Group 1986, 1993, 1996

First published 1986
Reprinted 1989
Reprinted 1990
Reprinted 1991
Second edition 1993
Reprinted 1994
Third edition 1996
Reprinted 2000
Fourth edition 2002

by the BMJ Publishing Group, BMA House, Tavistock Square,
London WC1H 9JR

British Library Cataloguing in Publication Data
A catalogue record for this book is available from the British Library

ISBN 0-7279-1518-5

Typeset by Newgen Imaging Systems (P) Ltd., Chennai, India
Printed in Malaysia by Times Offset

Cover image: Lumbar spine. Coloured *x* ray of four lumbar
vertebrae of the human spine, seen in antero-posterior view.
Reproduced with permission from Science Photo Library.

Contents

Contributors

Elizabeth Binks
Senior Sister, The Duke of Cornwall Spinal Treatment Centre, Salisbury District Hospital

John Carvell
Consultant Orthopaedic Surgeon, Salisbury District Hospital

Sue Cox Martin
Senior Occupational Therapist, The Duke of Cornwall Spinal Treatment Centre, Salisbury District Hospital

Peter Guy
Consultant Urologist, Salisbury District Hospital

John Hobby
Consultant Plastic Surgeon, Salisbury District Hospital

Julia Ingram
Social Worker, The Duke of Cornwall Spinal Treatment Centre, Salisbury District Hospital

Firas Jamil
Consultant in Spinal Injuries, The Duke of Cornwall Spinal Treatment Centre, Salisbury District Hospital

Andrew Morris
Consultant Radiologist, Salisbury District Hospital

Nigel North
Consultant Clinical Psychologist, The Duke of Cornwall Spinal Treatment Centre, Salisbury District Hospital

Wendy Pickard
Pressure Nurse Specialist, The Duke of Cornwall Spinal Treatment Centre, Salisbury District Hospital

Anba Soopramanien
Consultant in Spinal Injuries, The Duke of Cornwall Spinal Treatment Centre, Salisbury District Hospital

Rachel Stowell
Community Liaison Sister, The Duke of Cornwall Spinal Treatment Centre, Salisbury District Hospital

Ian Swain
Professor of Medical Physics and Bioengineering, Salisbury District Hospital

Anthony Tromans
Consultant in Spinal Injuries, The Duke of Cornwall Spinal Treatment Centre, Salisbury District Hospital

Trudy Ward
Therapy Manager, The Duke of Cornwall Spinal Treatment Centre, Salisbury District Hospital

Catriona Wood
Senior Clinical Nurse, The Duke of Cornwall Spinal Treatment Centre, Salisbury District Hospital

Preface

The fourth edition of the ABC of Spinal Cord Injury, although now redesigned in the current ABC style, has the same goals as previous editions. It assumes spinal cord injury to be the underlying condition, and it must be remembered that a slightly different approach is used for trauma patients in whom spinal column injury cannot be excluded but cord damage is not suspected.

This ABC aims to present in as clear a way as possible the correct management of patients with acute spinal cord injury, step by step, through all the phases of care and rehabilitation until eventual return to the community.

The book discusses how to move the injured patient from the scene of the accident, in conformity with pre-hospital techniques used by ambulance services in developed countries, and it incorporates refinements in advanced trauma life support (ATLS) which have developed over the past decade.

The text explains how to assess the patient, using updated information on the classification and neurological assessment of spinal cord injury.

There is a greater emphasis in making the correct diagnosis of spinal injury and established cord injury—unfortunately, litigation due to missed diagnosis is not uncommon. The pitfalls in diagnosis are identified, and by following the step by step approach described, failure to diagnose these serious injuries should therefore be minimised.

Patients with an acute spinal cord injury often have associated injuries, and the principles involved in managing these injuries are also discussed.

The later chapters follow the patient through the various stages of rehabilitation, and describe the specialised nursing, physiotherapy and occupational therapy required. They also discuss the social and psychological support needed for many of these patients in helping both patient and family adjust to what is often a lifetime of disability. Where applicable, the newer surgical advances, including the use of implants which can result in enhanced independence and mobility, are described.

Later complications and their management are discussed, and for the first time there is a chapter on the special challenges of managing spinal cord injuries in developing countries, where the incidence is higher and financial resources poorer than in the developed world.

David Grundy
Andrew Swain

1   At the accident

Andrew Swain, David Grundy

Spinal cord injury is a mortal condition and has been recognised as such since antiquity. In about 2500 BC, in the Edwin Smith papyrus, an unknown Egyptian physician accurately described the clinical features of traumatic tetraplegia (quadriplegia) and revealed an awareness of the awful prognosis with the chilling advice: "an ailment not to be treated". That view prevailed until the early years of this century. In the First World War 90% of patients who suffered a spinal cord injury died within one year of wounding and only about 1% survived more than 20 years. Fortunately, the vision of a few pioneers—Guttmann in the United Kingdom together with Munro and Bors in the United States—has greatly improved the outlook for those with spinal cord injury, although the mortality associated with tetraplegia was still 35% in the 1960s. The better understanding and management of spinal cord injury have led to a reduction in mortality and a higher incidence of incomplete spinal cord damage in those who survive. Ideal management now demands immediate evacuation from the scene of the accident to a centre where intensive care of the patient can be undertaken in liaison with a specialist in spinal cord injuries.

At present the annual incidence of spinal cord injury within the United Kingdom is about 10 to 15 per million of the population. In recent years there has been an increase in the proportion of injuries to the cervical spinal cord, and this is now the most common indication for admission to a spinal injuries unit.

Only about 5% of spinal cord injuries occur in children, mainly following road trauma or falls from a height greater than their own, but they sustain a complete cord injury more frequently than adults.

Although the effect of the initial trauma is irreversible, the spinal cord is at risk from further injury by injudicious early management. The emergency services must avoid such complications in unconscious patients by being aware of the possibility of spinal cord injury from the nature of the accident, and in conscious patients by suspecting the diagnosis from the history and basic examination. If such an injury is suspected the patient must be handled correctly from the outset.

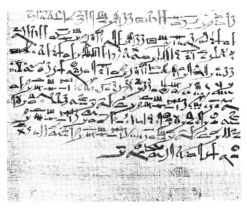

Figure 1.1 Edwin Smith papyrus. Reproduced with permission from Hughes JT. The Edwin Smith Papyrus. *Paraplegia* 1988:**26**:71–82.

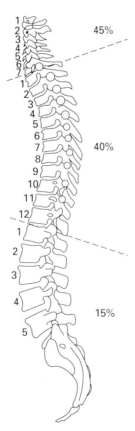

Figure 1.2 Proportion of cervical, thoracic, and lumbar injuries in 126 patients with spinal cord trauma admitted to the Duke of Cornwall Spinal Treatment Centre, 1997–99.

Box 1.1 Causes of spinal cord injury—126 new patient admissions to Duke of Cornwall Spinal Treatment Centre, 1997–99

Road traffic accidents	**45%**	**Domestic and industrial**	**34%**
Car, van, coach, lorry	16.5%	**accidents**	
Motorcycle	20%	Domestic—e.g. falls down	
Cycle	5.5%	stairs or from trees	
Pedestrian	1.5%	or ladders	22%
Aeroplane, helicopter	1.5%	Accidents at work—e.g.	
		falls from scaffolding or	
Self harm and criminal	**6%**	ladders, crush injuries	12%
assault			
Self harm	5%	**Injuries at sport**	**15%**
Criminal assault	1%	Diving into shallow water	4%
		Rugby	1%
		Horse riding	3%
		Miscellaneous—e.g.	
		gymnastics, motocross,	
		skiing, etc,	7%

Management at the scene of the accident

Doctors may witness or attend the scene of an accident, particularly if the casualty is trapped. Spinal injuries most commonly result from road trauma involving vehicles that overturn, unrestrained or ejected occupants, and motorcyclists. Falls from a height, high velocity crashes, and certain types of sports injury (e.g. diving into shallow water, collapse of a rugby scrum) should also raise immediate concern. Particular care must be taken moving unconscious patients, those who complain of pain in the back or neck, and those who describe altered sensation or loss of power in the limbs. Impaired consciousness (from injury or alcohol) and distracting injuries in multiple trauma are amongst the commonest causes of a failure to diagnose spinal injury. All casualties in the above risk categories should be assumed to have unstable spinal injuries until proven otherwise by a thorough examination and adequate x rays.

Spinal injuries involve more than one level in about 10% of cases. It must also be remembered that spinal cord injury without radiological abnormality (SCIWORA) can occur, and may be due to ligamentous damage with instability, or other soft tissue injuries such as traumatic central disc prolapse. SCIWORA is more common in children.

The unconscious patient

It must be assumed that the force that rendered the patient unconscious has injured the cervical spine until radiography of its entire length proves otherwise. Until then the head and neck must be carefully placed and held in the neutral (anatomical) position and stabilised. A rescuer can be delegated to perform this task throughout. However, splintage is best achieved with a rigid collar of appropriate size supplemented with sandbags or bolsters on each side of the head. The sandbags are held in position by tapes placed across the forehead and collar. If gross spinal deformity is left uncorrected and splinted, the cervical cord may sustain further injury from unrelieved angulation or compression. Alignment must be corrected unless attempts to do this increase pain or exacerbate neurological symptoms, or the head is locked in a position of torticollis (as in atlanto-axial rotatory subluxation). In these situations, the head must be splinted in the position found.

Thoracolumbar injury must also be assumed and treated by carefully straightening the trunk and correcting rotation. During turning or lifting, it is vital that the *whole* spine is maintained in the neutral position. While positioning the patient, relevant information can be obtained from witnesses and a brief assessment of superficial wounds may suggest the mechanism of injury—for example, wounds of the forehead often accompany hyperextension injuries of the cervical spine.

Although the spine is best immobilised by placing the patient supine, and this position is important for resuscitation and the rapid assessment of life threatening injuries, unconscious patients on their backs are at risk of passive gastric regurgitation and aspiration of vomit. This can be avoided by tracheal intubation, which is the ideal method of securing the airway in an unconscious casualty. If intubation cannot be performed the patient should be "log rolled" carefully into a modified lateral position 70–80° from prone with the head supported in the neutral position by the underlying arm. This posture allows secretions to drain freely from the mouth, and a rigid collar applied before the log roll helps to minimise neck movement. However, the position is unstable and therefore

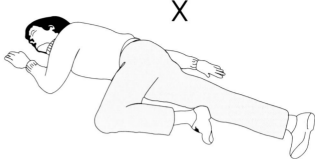

(a) Coma position—note that the spine is rotated.

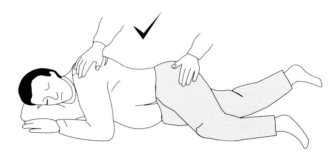

(b) Lateral position—two hands from a rescuer stabilise the shoulder and left upper thigh to prevent the patient from falling forwards or backwards.

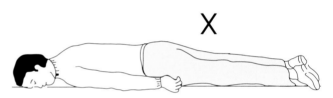

(c) Prone position—compromises respiration.

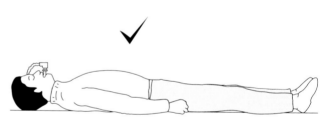

(d) Supine position—if patient is supine the airway must be secure, and if consciousness is impaired, the patient should be intubated.

Figure 1.3 Positions.

needs to be maintained by a rescuer. Log rolling should ideally be performed by a minimum of four people in a coordinated manner, ensuring that unnecessary movement does not occur in any part of the spine. During this manoeuvre, the team leader will move the patient's head through an arc as it rotates with the rest of the body.

The prone position is unsatisfactory as it may severely embarrass respiration, particularly in the tetraplegic patient. The original semiprone coma position is also contraindicated, as it results in rotation of the neck. Modifications of the latter position are taught on first aid and cardiopulmonary resuscitation courses where the importance of airway maintenance and ease of positioning overrides that of cervical alignment, particularly for bystanders.

Patency of the airway and adequate oxygenation must take priority in unconscious patients. If the casualty is wearing a one-piece full-face helmet, access to the airway is achieved using a two-person technique: one rescuer immobilises the neck from below whilst the other pulls the sides of the helmet outwards and slides them over the ears. On some modern helmets, release buttons allow the face piece to hinge upwards and expose the mouth. After positioning the casualty and immobilising the neck, the mouth should be opened by jaw thrust or chin lift without head tilt. Any intra-oral debris can then be cleared before an oropharyngeal airway is sized and inserted, and high concentration oxygen given.

The indications for tracheal intubation in spinal injury are similar to those for other trauma patients: the presence of an insecure airway or inadequate arterial oxygen saturation (i.e. less than 90%) despite the administration of high concentrations of oxygen. With care, intubation is usually safe in patients with injuries to the spinal cord, and may be performed at the scene of the accident or later in the hospital receiving room, depending on the patient's level of consciousness and the ability of the attending doctor or paramedic. Orotracheal intubation is rendered more safe if an assistant holds the head and minimises neck movement and the procedure may be facilitated by using an intubation bougie. Other specialised airway devices such as the laryngeal mask airway (LMA) or Combitube may be used but each has its limitations—for example the former device does not prevent aspiration and use of the latter device requires training.

If possible, suction should be avoided in tetraplegic patients as it may stimulate the vagal reflex, aggravate preexisting bradycardia, and occasionally precipitate cardiac arrest (to be discussed later). The risk of unwanted vagal effects can be minimised if atropine and oxygen are administered beforehand. In hospital, flexible fibreoptic instruments may provide the ideal solution to the intubation of patients with cervical fractures or dislocations.

Once the airway is protected intravenous access should be established as multiple injuries frequently accompany spinal cord trauma. However, clinicians should remember that in uncomplicated cases of high spinal cord injury (cervical and upper thoracic), patients may be hypotensive due to sympathetic paralysis and may easily be overinfused.

If respiration and circulation are satisfactory patients can be examined briefly where they lie or in an ambulance. A basic examination should include measurement of respiratory rate, pulse, and blood pressure; brief assessment of the level of consciousness and pupillary responses; and examination of the head, chest, abdomen, pelvis and limbs for obvious signs of trauma. Diaphragmatic breathing due to intercostal paralysis may be seen in patients with tetraplegia or high thoracic paraplegia, and flaccidity with areflexia may be present in the paralysed limbs. If the casualty's back is easily exposed, spinal deformity or an increased interspinous gap may be identified.

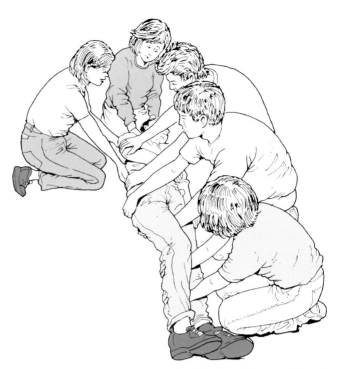

Figure 1.4 Deployment of personnel and hand positions used when log rolling a patient from the supine to the lateral position. The person on the left is free to inspect the back.

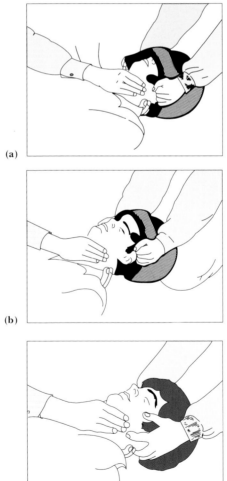

(a)

(b)

(c)

Figure 1.5 Safe removal of a full-face helmet requires two rescuers. One immobilises the neck in the neutral position from below using two hands whilst the other removes the jaw strap, spreads the lateral margins of the helmet apart, and gently eases the helmet upwards. Tilting the helmet forwards helps to avoid flexion of the neck as the occiput rides over the posterior lip of the helmet but care must be taken not to trap the nose.

The conscious patient

The diagnosis of spinal cord injury rests on the symptoms and signs of pain in the spine, sensory disturbance, and weakness or flaccid paralysis. In conscious patients with these features resuscitative measures should again be given priority. At the same time a brief history can be obtained, which will help to localise the level of spinal trauma and identify other injuries that may further compromise the nutrition of the damaged spinal cord by producing hypoxia or hypovolaemic shock. The patient must be made to lie down—some have been able to walk a short distance before becoming paralysed—and the supine position prevents orthostatic hypotension. A brief general examination should be undertaken at the scene and a basic neurological assessment made by asking patients to what extent they can feel or move their limbs.

Analgesia

In the acute phase of injury, control of the patient's pain is important, especially if multiple trauma has occurred. Analgesia is initially best provided by intravenous opioids titrated slowly until comfort is achieved. Opioids should be used with caution when cervical or upper thoracic spinal cord injuries have been sustained and ventilatory function may already be impaired. Naloxone must be available. Careful monitoring of consciousness, respiratory rate and depth, and oxygen saturation can give warning of respiratory depression.

Intramuscular or rectal non-steroidal anti-inflammatory drugs are effective in providing background analgesia.

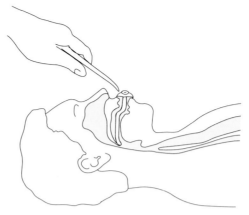

Figure 1.6 Suction: beware of vagal reflex stimulation and bradycardia.

> **Box 1.2 Clinical features of spinal cord injury**
>
> - **Pain in the neck or back, often radiating because of nerve root irritation**
> - **Sensory disturbance distal to neurological level**
> - **Weakness or flaccid paralysis below this level**

> **Opioid analgesics should be administered with care in patients with respiratory compromise from cervical and upper thoracic injuries**

Further reading

- Go BK, DeVivo MJ, Richards JS. The epidemiology of spinal cord injury. In: Stover SL, DeLisa JA, Whiteneck GG, eds. *Spinal cord injury. Clinical outcomes from the model systems.* Gaithersburg: Aspen Publishers, 1995, pp 21–55
- Greaves I, Porter KM. *Prehospital medicine.* London: Arnold, 1999
- Swain A. Trauma to the spine and spinal cord. In: Skinner D, Swain A, Peyton R, Robertson C, eds. *Cambridge textbook of accident and emergency medicine.* Cambridge: Cambridge University Press, 1997, pp 510–32
- Toscano J. Prevention of neurological deterioration before admission to a spinal cord injury unit. *Paraplegia* 1988;**26**:143–50

2 Evacuation and initial management at hospital

Andrew Swain, David Grundy

Evacuation and transfer to hospital

In the absence of an immediate threat to life such as fire, collapsing masonry, or cardiac arrest, casualties at risk of spinal injury should be positioned on a spinal board or immobiliser before they are moved from the position in which they were initially found. Immobilisers are short backboards that can be applied to a patient sitting in a car seat whilst the head and neck are supported in the neutral position. In some cases the roof of the vehicle is removed or the back seat is lowered to allow a full-length spinal board to be slid under the patient from the rear of the vehicle. A long board can also be inserted obliquely under the patient through an open car door, but this requires coordination and training as the casualty has to be carefully rotated on the board without twisting the spine, and then be laid back into the supine position. Spinal immobilisers do not effectively splint the pelvis or lumbar spine but they can be left in place whilst the patient is transferred to a long board.

Both short and long back splints must be used in conjunction with a semirigid collar of appropriate size to prevent movement of the upper spine. If the correct collars or splints are not available manual immobilisation of the head is the safest option. Small children can be splinted to a child seat with good effect—padding is placed as necessary between the head and the side cushions and forehead strapping can then be applied.

If lying free, the casualty should ideally be turned by four people: one responsible for the head and neck, one for the shoulders and chest, one for the hips and abdomen, and one for the legs. The person holding the head and neck directs movement. This team can work together to align the spine in a neutral position and then perform a log roll allowing a spinal board to be placed under the patient. Alternatively the patient can be transferred to a spinal board using a "scoop" stretcher which can be carefully slotted together around the casualty.

In the flexion-extension axis, the neutral position of the cervical spine varies with the age of the patient. The relatively large head and prominent occiput of small children (less than 8 years of age) pushes their neck into flexion when they lie on a flat surface. This is corrected on paediatric spinal boards by thoracic padding, which elevates the back and restores neutral curvature. Conversely, elderly patients may have a thoracic kyphosis and for this a pillow needs to be inserted between the occiput and the adult spinal board if the head is not to fall back into hyperextension. In all instances, the aim is to achieve normal cervical curvature for the individual. For example, extension should not be enforced on a patient with fixed cervical flexion attributable to ankylosing spondylitis.

A small child may not tolerate a backboard. One alternative is a vacuum splint (adult lower limb size) which can be wrapped around the child like a vacuum mattress (see below). However, an uncooperative or distressed child might have to be carried by a paramedic or parent in as neutral a position as possible, and be comforted en route.

For transportation, the patient should be supine if conscious or intubated. In the unconscious patient whose airway cannot be protected, the lateral or head-down positions are safer and these can be achieved by tilting or turning the patient who must be strapped to the spinal board. To stabilise the neck on the spinal board, the semirigid collar must be

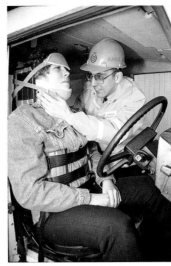

Figure 2.1 Patient being removed from a vehicle with a semirigid collar and spinal immobiliser (Kendrick extrication device) in position.

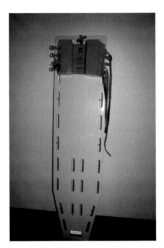

Figure 2.2 Spinal board with head bolsters and straps.

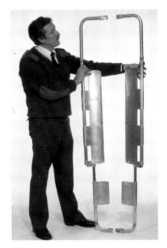

Figure 2.3 Scoop stretcher.

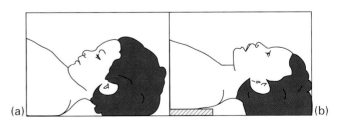

Figure 2.4 Cervical flexion on a spinal board attributable to the relatively prominent occiput that is characteristic of smaller children (a). The flexion can be relieved by inserting padding under the thoracic spine (b).

supplemented with sandbags or bolsters taped to the forehead and collar. Only the physically uncooperative or thrashing patient is exempt from full splintage of the head and neck as this patient may manipulate the cervical spine from below if the head and neck are fixed in position. In this circumstance, the patient should be fitted with a semirigid collar only and be encouraged to lie still. Such uncooperative behaviour should not be attributed automatically to alcohol, as hypoxia and shock may be responsible and must be treated.

If no spinal board is used and the airway is unprotected, the modified lateral position (Figure 1.3(b)) is recommended with the spine neutral and the body held in position by a rescuer. In the absence of life-threatening injury, patients with spinal injury should be transported smoothly by ambulance, for reasons of comfort as well as to avoid further trauma to the spinal cord. They should be taken to the nearest major emergency department but must be repeatedly assessed en route; in particular, vital functions must be monitored. In transit the head and neck must be maintained in the neutral position at all times. If an unintubated supine trauma patient starts to vomit, it is safer to tip the casualty head down and apply oropharyngeal suction than to attempt an uncoordinated turn into the lateral position. However, patients can be turned safely and rapidly by a single rescuer when strapped to a spinal board and that is one of the advantages of this device.

Hard objects should be removed from patients' pockets during transit, and anaesthetic areas should be protected to prevent pressure sores.

The usual vasomotor responses to changes of temperature are impaired in tetraplegia and high paraplegia because the sympathetic system is paralysed. The patient is therefore poikilothermic, and hypothermia is a particular risk when these patients are transported during the winter months. A warm environment, blankets, and thermal reflector sheets help to maintain body temperature.

When the patient has been injured in an inaccessible location or has to be evacuated over a long distance, transfer by helicopter has been shown to reduce mortality and morbidity. If a helicopter is used, the possibility of immediate transfer to a regional spinal injuries unit with acute support facilities should be considered after discussion with that unit.

Initial management at the receiving hospital

Primary survey

When the patient arrives at the nearest major emergency department, a detailed history must be obtained from ambulance staff, witnesses, and if possible the patient. Simultaneously, the patient is transferred to the trauma trolley and this must be expeditious but smooth. If the patient is attached to a spinal board, this is an ideal transfer device and resuscitation can continue on the spinal board with only momentary interruption. Alternatively a scoop stretcher can be used for the transfer but this will take longer. In the absence of either device, the patient can be subjected to a coordinated spinal lift but this requires training.

A full general and neurological assessment must be undertaken in accordance with the principles of advanced trauma life support (ATLS). The examination must be thorough because spinal trauma is frequently associated with multiple injuries. As always, the patient's airway, breathing and circulation ("ABC"—in that order) are the first priorities in

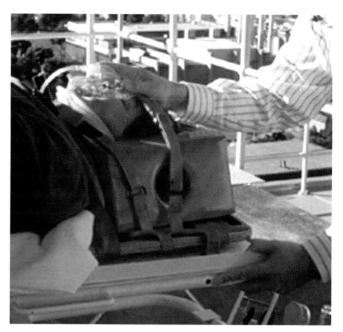

Figure 2.5 Patient on spinal board—close-up view to show the semirigid collar, bolsters and positioning of the straps.

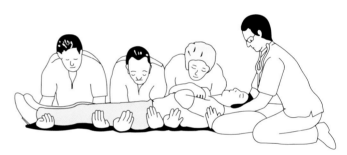

Figure 2.6 A coordinated spinal lift.

Box 2.1 Associated injuries—new injury admissions to Duke of Cornwall Spinal Treatment Centre 1997–99

Spinal cord injury is accompanied by:
Head injuries (coma of more than 6 hours' duration,
  brain contusion or skull fracture)   in 12%
Chest injuries (requiring active treatment,
  or rib fractures)   in 19%
Abdominal injuries (requiring laparotomy)   in 3%
Limb injuries   in 20%

resuscitation from trauma. If not already secure, the cervical spine is immobilised in the neutral position as the airway is assessed. Following attention to the ABC, a central nervous system assessment is undertaken and any clothing is removed. This sequence constitutes the primary survey of ATLS. The spinal injury itself can directly affect the airway (for example by producing a retropharyngeal haematoma or tracheal deviation) as well as the respiratory and circulatory systems (see chapter 4).

Secondary survey

Once the immediately life-threatening injuries have been addressed, the secondary (head to toe) survey that follows allows other serious injuries to be identified. Areas that are not being examined should be covered and kept warm, and body temperature should be monitored. In the supine position, the cervical and lumbar lordoses may be palpated by sliding a hand under the patient. A more comprehensive examination is made during the log roll. Unless there is an urgent need to inspect the back, the log roll is normally undertaken near the end of the secondary survey by a team of four led by the person who holds the patient's head. If neurological symptoms or signs are present, a senior doctor should be present and a partial roll to about 45° may be sufficient. A doctor who is not involved with the log roll must examine the back for specific signs of injury including local bruising or deformity of the spine (e.g. a gibbus or an increased interspinous gap) and vertebral tenderness. The whole length of the spine must be palpated, as about 10% of patients with an unstable spinal injury have another spinal injury at a different level. Priapism and diaphragmatic breathing invariably indicate a high spinal cord lesion. The presence of warm and well-perfused peripheries in a hypotensive patient should always raise the possibility of neurogenic shock attributable to spinal cord injury in the

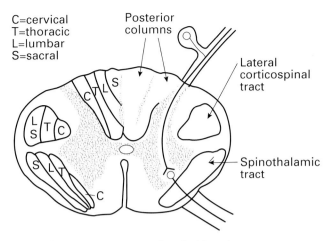

Figure 2.7 Cross-section of spinal cord, with main tracts.

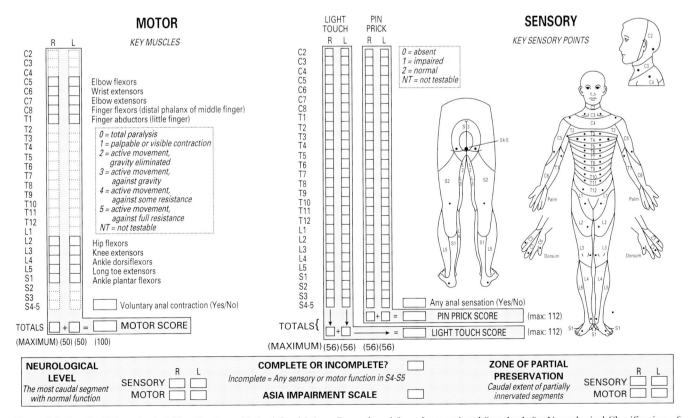

Figure 2.8 Standard Neurological Classification of Spinal Cord Injury. Reproduced from International Standards for Neurological Classification of Spinal Cord Injury, revised 2000. American Spinal Injury Association/International Medical Society of Paraplegia.

differential diagnosis. At the end of the secondary survey, examination of the peripheral nervous system must not be neglected.

The log roll during the secondary survey provides an ideal opportunity to remove the spinal board from the patient. It has been demonstrated that high pressure exists at the interfaces between the board and the occiput, scapulae, sacrum, and heels. It is generally recommended that the spinal board is removed within 30 minutes of its application whenever possible. The head and neck can then be splinted to the trauma trolley. If full splintage is required following removal of the spinal board, especially for transit between hospitals, use of a vacuum mattress is recommended. This device is contoured to the patient before air is evacuated from it with a pump. The vacuum causes the plastic beads within the mattress to lock into position. Interface pressures are much lower when a vacuum mattress is used and patients find the device much more comfortable than a spinal board. Paediatric vacuum mattresses are also available and they may be used at the accident scene.

A specific clinical problem in spinal cord injury is the early diagnosis of intra-abdominal trauma during the secondary survey. This may be very difficult in patients with high cord lesions (above the seventh thoracic segment) during the initial phase of spinal shock, when paralytic ileus and abdominal distension are usual. Abdominal sensation is impaired, and this, together with the flaccid paralysis, means that the classical features of an intra-abdominal emergency may be absent. The signs of peritoneal irritation do not develop but pain may be referred to the shoulder from the diaphragm and this is an important symptom. When blunt abdominal trauma is suspected, peritoneal lavage or computed tomography is recommended unless clinical concern justifies immediate laparotomy. Abdominal bruising from seat belts, especially isolated lap belts in children, is associated with injuries to the bowel, pancreas and lumbar spine.

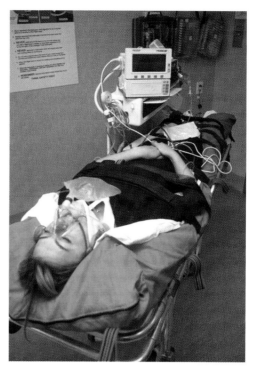

Figure 2.9 Patient on a vacuum mattress. For secure immobilisation during transportation, forehead and collar tapes should be applied.

Neurological assessment

In spinal cord injury the neurological examination must include assessment of the following:

- Sensation to pin prick (spinothalamic tracts)
- Sensation to fine touch and joint position sense (posterior columns)
- Power of muscle groups according to the Medical Research Council scale (corticospinal tracts)
- Reflexes (including abdominal, anal, and bulbocavernosus)
- Cranial nerve function (may be affected by high cervical injury, e.g. dysphagia).

By examining the dermatomes and myotomes in this way, the level and completeness of the spinal cord injury and the presence of other neurological damage such as brachial plexus injury are assessed. The last segment of normal spinal cord function, as judged by clinical examination, is referred to as the neurological level of the lesion. This does not necessarily correspond with the level of bony injury (Figure 5.1), so the neurological and bony diagnoses should both be recorded. Sensory or motor sparing may be present below the injury.

Traditionally, incomplete spinal cord lesions have been defined as those in which some sensory or motor function is preserved below the level of neurological injury. The American Spinal Injury Association (ASIA) has now produced the ASIA impairment scale modified from the Frankel grades (see page 74). Incomplete injuries have been redefined as those

Box 2.2 Diagnosis of intra-abdominal trauma often difficult because of:

- impaired or absent abdominal sensation
- absent abdominal guarding or rigidity, because of flaccid paralysis
- paralytic ileus

Box 2.3 If blunt abdominal trauma suspected

- peritoneal lavage
- abdominal CT scan with contrast

associated with some preservation of sensory or motor function below the neurological level, including the lowest sacral segment. This is determined by the presence of sensation both superficially at the mucocutaneous junction and deeply within the anal canal, or alternatively by intact voluntary contraction of the external anal sphincter on digital examination. ASIA also describes the zone of partial preservation (ZPP) which refers to the dermatomes and myotomes that remain partially innervated below the main neurological level. The exact number of segments so affected should be recorded for both sides of the body. The term ZPP is used only with injuries that do not satisfy the ASIA definition of "incomplete".

ASIA has produced a form incorporating these definitions (Figure 2.8). The muscles tested by ASIA are chosen because of the consistency of their nerve supply by the segments indicated, and because they can all be tested with the patient in the supine position.

ASIA also states that other muscles should be evaluated, but their grades are not used in determining the motor score and level. The muscles not listed on the ASIA Standard Neurological Classification form, with their nerve supply, are as follows:

Diaphragm—C3,4,5
Shoulder abductors—C5
Supinators/pronators—C6
Wrist flexors—C7
Finger extensors—C7
Intrinsic hand muscles—T1
Hip adductors—L2,3
Knee flexors—L4,5 S1
Toe flexors—S1,2.

Spinal shock

After severe spinal cord injury, generalised flaccidity below the level of the lesion supervenes, but it is rare for all reflexes to be absent in the first few weeks except in lower motor neurone lesions. The classical description of spinal shock as the period following injury during which all spinal reflexes are absent should therefore be discarded, particularly as almost a third of patients examined within 1–3 hours of injury have reflexes present.

The delayed plantar response (DPR) is present in all patients with complete injuries. It is demonstrated by pressing firmly with a blunt instrument from the heel toward the toes along the lateral sole of the foot and continuing medially across the volar aspect of the metatarsal heads. Following the stimulus the toes flex and relax in delayed sequence. The flexion component can be misinterpreted as a normal plantar response.

The deep tendon reflexes are more predictable: usually absent in complete cord lesions, and present in the majority of patients with incomplete injuries.

The anal and bulbocavernosus reflexes both depend on intact sacral reflex arcs. The anal reflex is an externally visible contraction of the anal sphincter in response to perianal pin prick. The bulbocavernosus reflex is a similar contraction of the anal sphincter felt with the examining finger in response to squeezing the glans penis. They may aid in distinguishing between an upper motor neurone lesion, in which the reflex may not return for several days, and a lower motor neurone lesion, in which the reflex remains ablated unless neurological recovery occurs. Examples of such lower motor neurone lesions are injuries to the conus and cauda equina.

Box 2.4 Reflexes and their nerve supply

Biceps jerk	C5,6
Supinator jerk	C6
Triceps jerk	C7
Abdominal reflex	T8–12
Knee jerk	L3,4
Ankle jerk	L5,S1
Bulbocavernosus reflex	S3,4
Anal reflex	S5
Plantar reflex	

Spinal reflexes after cord injury

Note:
Almost one third of patients with spinal cord injury examined within 1–3 hours of injury have reflexes

---

Plantar reflex after cord injury

Distinguish between:
- **Delayed plantar response—present in all complete injuries**
- **Normal plantar response**

Box 2.5 ASIA Impairment Scale—used in grading the degree of impairment

A = Complete. No sensory or motor function is preserved in the sacral segments S4–S5
B = Incomplete. Sensory but not motor function is preserved below the neurological level and extends through the sacral segments S4–S5
C = Incomplete. Motor function is preserved below the neurological level, and the majority of key muscles below the neurological level have a muscle grade less than 3
D = Incomplete. Motor function is preserved below the neurological level, and the majority of key muscles below the neurological level have a muscle grade greater than or equal to 3
E = Normal. Sensory and motor function is normal

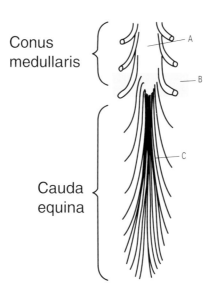

Figure 2.10 Conus medullaris and Cauda equina syndromes. (Reproduced with permission from Maynard FM *et al. Spinal Cord* 1997;**35**:266–74.)

Partial spinal cord injury

Neurological symptoms and signs may not fit a classic pattern or demonstrate a clear neurological level. For this reason, some cord injuries are not infrequently misdiagnosed and attributed to hysterical or conversion paralysis. Neurological symptoms or signs must not be dismissed until spinal cord injury has been excluded by means of a thorough examination and appropriate clinical investigations.

Assessment of the level and completeness of the spinal cord injury allows a prognosis to be made. If the lesion is complete from the outset, recovery is far less likely than in an incomplete lesion.

Following trauma to the spinal cord and cauda equina there are recognised patterns of injury, and variations of these may present in the emergency department.

Anterior cord syndrome

The anterior part of the spinal cord is usually injured by a flexion-rotation force to the spine producing an anterior dislocation or by a compression fracture of the vertebral body with bony encroachment on the vertebral canal. There is often anterior spinal artery compression so that the corticospinal and spinothalamic tracts are damaged by a combination of direct trauma and ischaemia. This results in loss of power as well as reduced pain and temperature sensation below the lesion.

Central cord syndrome

This is typically seen in older patients with cervical spondylosis. A hyperextension injury, often from relatively minor trauma, compresses the spinal cord between the irregular osteophytic vertebral body and the intervertebral disc anteriorly and the thickened ligamentum flavum posteriorly. The more centrally situated cervical tracts supplying the arms suffer the brunt of the injury so that classically there is a flaccid (lower motor neurone) weakness of the arms and relatively strong but spastic (upper motor neurone) leg function. Sacral sensation and bladder and bowel function are often partially spared.

Posterior cord syndrome

This syndrome is most commonly seen in hyperextension injuries with fractures of the posterior elements of the vertebrae. There is contusion of the posterior columns so the patient may have good power and pain and temperature sensation but there is sometimes profound ataxia due to the loss of proprioception, which can make walking very difficult.

Brown–Séquard syndrome

Classically resulting from stab injuries but also common in lateral mass fractures of the vertebrae, the signs of the Brown-Séquard syndrome are those of a hemisection of the spinal cord. Power is reduced or absent but pain and temperature sensation are relatively normal on the side of the injury because the spinothalamic tract crosses over to the opposite side of the cord. The uninjured side therefore has good power but reduced or absent sensation to pin prick and temperature.

Conus medullaris syndrome

The effect of injury to the sacral cord (conus medullaris) and lumbar nerve roots (as at B, Figure 2.10) is usually loss of bladder, bowel and lower limb reflexes. Lesions high in the conus (as at A, Figure 2.10) may occasionally represent upper motor neurone defects and function may then be preserved in the sacral reflexes, for example the bulbocavernosus and micturition reflexes.

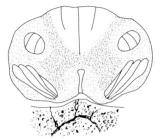

Anterior cord syndrome

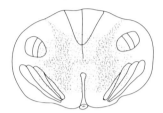

Central cord syndrome

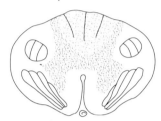

Posterior cord syndrome

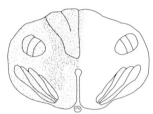

Brown–Séquard syndrome

Figure 2.11 Cross-sections of the spinal cord, showing partial spinal cord injury syndromes.

Cauda equina syndrome

Injury to the lumbosacral nerve roots (as at C, Figure 2.10) results in areflexia of the bladder, bowel, and lower limbs.

The final phase in the diagnosis of spinal trauma entails radiology of the spine to assess the level and nature of the injury.

Further reading

- *Advanced trauma life support program for doctors*, 6th edition. Chicago: American College of Surgeons, 1997
- Ko H-Y, Ditunno JF, Graziani V, Little JW. The pattern of reflex recovery during spinal shock. *Spinal Cord* 1999;**37**:402–9
- Main PW, Lovell ME. A review of seven support surfaces with emphasis on their protection of the spinally injured. *J Accid Emerg Med* 1996;**13**:34–7
- Maynard FM *et al*. International standards for neurological and functional classification of spinal cord injury. *Spinal Cord* 1997;**35**:266–74

3   Radiological investigations

David Grundy, Andrew Swain, Andrew Morris

Radiological investigation of a high standard is crucial to the diagnosis of a spinal injury. Initial radiographs are taken in the emergency department. Most emergency departments rely on the use of mobile radiographic equipment for investigating seriously ill patients, but the quality of films obtained in this way is usually inferior.

Once the patient's condition is stable, radiographs can be taken in the radiology department. In the presence of neurological symptoms, a doctor should be in attendance to ensure that any spinal movement is minimised. Sandbags and collars are not always radiolucent, and clearer radiographs may be obtained if these are removed after preliminary films have been taken. Plain x ray pictures in the lateral and anteroposterior projections are fundamental in the diagnosis of spinal injuries. Special views, computed tomography (CT), and magnetic resonance imaging (MRI) are used for further evaluation.

Spinal cord injury without radiological abnormality (SCIWORA) may occur due to central disc prolapse, ligamentous damage, or cervical spondylosis which narrows the spinal canal, makes it more rigid, and therefore renders the spinal cord more vulnerable to trauma (particularly in cervical hyperextension injuries). SCIWORA is also relatively common in injured children because greater mobility of the developing spine affords less protection to the spinal cord.

Cervical injuries

The first and most important spinal radiograph to be taken of a patient with a suspected cervical cord injury is the lateral view obtained with the x ray beam horizontal. This is much more likely than the anteroposterior view to show spinal damage and it can be taken in the emergency department without moving the supine patient. Other views are best obtained in the radiology department later. An anteroposterior radiograph and an open mouth view of the odontoid process must be taken to complete the basic series of cervical films but the latter normally requires removal of the collar and some adjustment of position, therefore the lateral x ray needs to be scrutinised first.

The lateral view should be repeated if the original radiograph does not show the whole of the cervical spine and the upper part of the first thoracic vertebra. Failure to insist on this often results in injuries of the lower cervical spine being missed. The lower cervical vertebrae are normally obscured by the shoulders unless these are depressed by traction on both arms. The traction must be stopped if it produces pain in the neck or exacerbates any neurological symptoms.

If the lower cervical spine is still not seen, a supine "swimmer's" view should be taken. With the near shoulder depressed and the arm next to the cassette abducted, abnormalities as far down as the first or second thoracic vertebra will usually be shown. This view is not easy to interpret, and does not produce clear bony detail (Figure 3.4), but it does provide an assessment of the alignment of the cervicothoracic junction. Oblique, supine views may also help in this situation.

The interpretation of cervical spine radiographs may pose problems for the inexperienced. First, remember that the spine consists of bones (visible) and soft tissues (invisible)

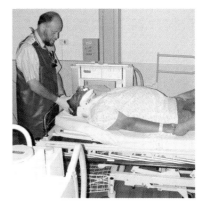

Figure 3.1 Lateral cervical spine radiograph being taken. Note traction on the arms.

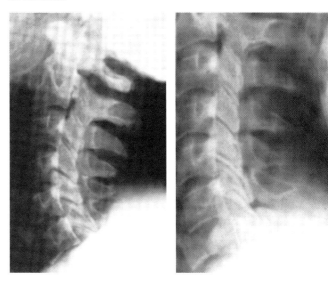

Figure 3.2 Compression fracture of C7, missed initially because of failure to show the entire cervical spine.

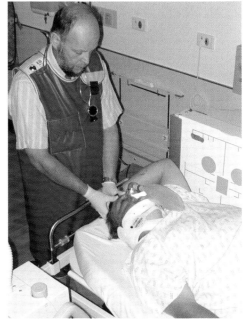

Figure 3.3 Swimmer's view being taken, with patient supine.

11

(Figure 3.6). These are functionally arranged into three columns, anterior, middle, and posterior, which together support the stability of the spine (Figure 3.13). Next assess the radiograph using the sequence ABCs.

"A" for alignment

Follow four lines on the lateral radiograph (Figure 3.7):

1. The fronts of the vertebral bodies—anterior longitudinal ligament.
2. The backs of the vertebral bodies—posterior longitudinal ligament.
3. The bases of the spinous processes (ligamentum flavum)— spinolaminar line.
4. The tips of the spinous processes.

The anterior arch of C1 lies in front of the odontoid process and is therefore anterior to the first line described (unless the odontoid is fractured and displaced posteriorly). Extended upwards, the spinolaminar line should cross the posterior margin of the foramen magnum. A line drawn downwards from the dorsum sellae along the surface of the clivus across the anterior margin of the foramen magnum should bisect the tip of the odontoid process.

"B" for bones

Follow the outline of each individual vertebra, and check for any steps or breaks.

"C" for cartilages

Examine the intervertebral discs and facet joints for displacement. The disc space may be widened if the annulus fibrosus is ruptured or narrowed in degenerative disc disease.

"S" for soft tissues

Check for widening of the soft tissues anterior to the spine on the lateral radiograph, denoting a prevertebral haematoma, and also widening of any bony interspaces indicating ligamentous damage—for instance separation of the spinous processes following damage to the interspinous and supraspinous ligaments posteriorly.

If the anterior or posterior displacement of one vertebra on another exceeds 3.5 mm on the lateral cervical radiograph, this must be considered abnormal. Anterior displacement of less than half the diameter of the vertebral body suggests unilateral facet dislocation; displacement greater than this indicates a bilateral facet dislocation. Atlanto-axial subluxation may be identified by an increased gap (more than 3 mm in adults and 5 mm in children) between the odontoid process and the anterior arch of the atlas on the lateral radiograph.

On the lateral radiograph, widening of the gap between adjacent spinous processes following rupture of the posterior cervical ligamentous complex denotes an unstable injury which is often associated with vertebral subluxation and a crush fracture of the vertebral body. The retropharyngeal space (at C2) should not exceed 7 mm in adults or children whereas the retrotracheal space (C6) should not be wider than 22 mm in adults or 14 mm in children (the retropharyngeal space widens in a crying child).

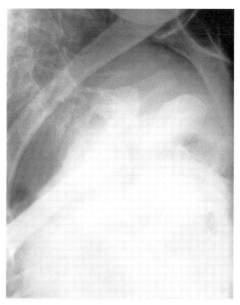

Figure 3.4 Swimmer's view—note the dislocation of C6–7 seen immediately below the clavicular shadow.

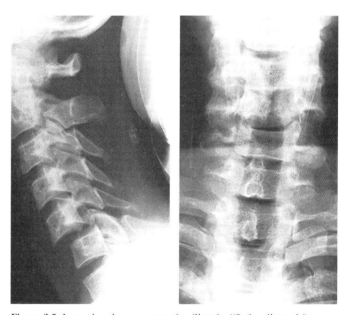

Figure 3.5 Lateral and anteroposterior films in C5–6 unilateral facet dislocation. Note the less-than-half vertebral body slip in the lateral view, and the lack of alignment of spinous processes, owing to rotation, in the anteroposterior view.

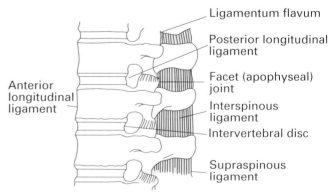

Figure 3.6 Spinal anatomy—lateral view.

Fractures of the anteroinferior margin of the vertebral body ("teardrop" fractures) are often associated with an unstable flexion injury and sometimes retropulsion of the vertebral body or disc material into the spinal canal. Similarly, flakes of bone may be avulsed from the anterosuperior margin of the vertebral body by the anterior longitudinal ligament in severe extension injuries.

On the anteroposterior radiograph, displacement of a spinous process from the midline may be explained by vertebral rotation secondary to unilateral facet dislocation, the spinous process being displaced towards the side of the dislocation. The spine is relatively stable in a unilateral facet dislocation, especially if maintained in extension. With a bilateral facet dislocation, the spinous processes are in line, the spine is always unstable, and the patient therefore requires extreme care when

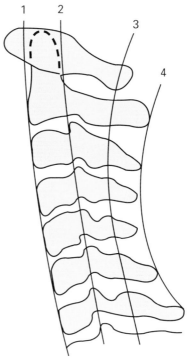

Figure 3.7 Lines of alignment on lateral radiograph.

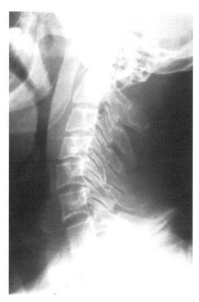

Figure 3.8 Lateral radiograph of cervical spine demonstrating prevertebral swelling in the upper cervical region in the absence of any obvious fracture. Other views confirmed a fracture of C2.

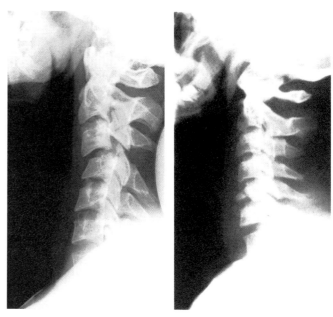

Figure 3.9 Left: C3–4 dislocation, postreduction film showing continuing instability because of posterior ligamentous damage. Right: teardrop fracture of C5 with retropulsion of vertebral body into spinal canal.

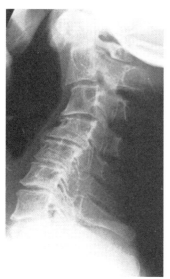
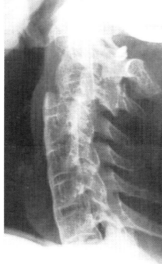

Figure 3.10 Left: central cord syndrome without bony damage, in a patient with cervical spondylosis. Right: transverse fracture through C3 in a patient with ankylosing spondylitis.

being handled. The anteroposterior cervical radiograph also provides an opportunity to examine the upper thoracic vertebrae and first to third ribs: severe trauma is required to injure these structures.

Oblique radiographs are not routinely obtained, but they do help to confirm the presence of subluxation or dislocation and indicate whether the right or left facets (apophyseal joints), or both, are affected. They may elucidate abnormalities at the cervicothoracic junction and some authorities recommend them as part of a five-view cervical spine series.

The 45° supine oblique view shows the intervertebral foramina and the facets but a better view for the facets is one taken with the patient log rolled 22.5° from the horizontal.

Flexion and extension views of the cervical spine may be taken if the patient has no neurological symptoms or signs and initial radiographs are normal but an unstable (ligamentous) injury is nevertheless suspected from the mechanism of injury, severe pain, or radiological signs of ligamentous injury. To obtain these radiographs, flexion and extension of the whole neck must be performed as far as the patient can tolerate under the supervision of an experienced doctor. Movement must cease if neurological symptoms are precipitated.

If there is any doubt about the integrity of the cervical spine on plain radiographs, CT should be performed. This provides much greater detail of the bony structures and will show the extent of encroachment on the spinal canal by vertebral displacement or bone fragments. It is particularly useful in assessing the cervicothoracic junction, the upper cervical spine and any suspected fracture or misalignment. Helical (or spiral) CT is now more available. It allows for a faster examination and also clearer reconstructed images in the sagittal and coronal planes. Many patients with major trauma will require CT of their head, chest or abdomen, and it is often appropriate to scan any suspicious or poorly seen area of their spine at the same time rather than struggle with further plain films.

MRI gives information about the spinal cord and soft tissues and will reveal the cause of cord compression, whether from bone, prolapsed discs, ligamentous damage, or intraspinal haematomas. It will also show the extent of cord damage and oedema which is of some prognostic value. Although an acute traumatic disc prolapse may be associated with bony injury, it can also occur with normal radiographs, and in these patients it is vital that an urgent MRI scan is obtained. These scans can also be used to demonstrate spinal instability, particularly in the presence of normal radiographs. MRI has superseded myelography, both in the quality of images obtained and in safety for the patient, allowing decisions to be made without the need for invasive imaging modalities. Its use may be limited by its availability and the difficulty in monitoring the acutely injured patient within the scanner.

Pathological changes in the spine—for example, ankylosing spondylitis or rheumatoid arthritis—may predispose to bony damage after relatively minor trauma and in these patients further radiological investigation and imaging must be thorough.

Thoracic and lumbar injuries

The thoracic spine is often demonstrated well on the anteroposterior chest radiograph that forms part of the standard series of views requested in major trauma. This *x* ray may be the first to reveal an injury to the thoracic spine. Radiographs of the thoracic and lumbar spine must be specifically requested if a cervical spine injury has been

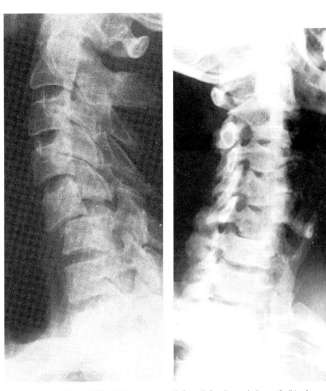

Figure 3.11 The 22.5° oblique view of the right facet joints (left) shows clearly the facet dislocation at the C5–6 level, less obvious in the 45° oblique view (right), which, however, shows a malalignment of the intervertebral foramina.

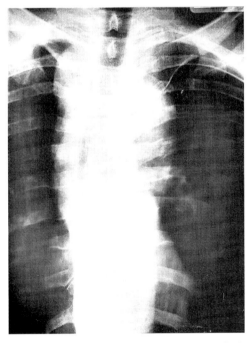

Figure 3.12 Patient with fracture of T5 with widening of mediastinum due to a prevertebral haematoma, initially diagnosed as traumatic dissection of the aorta, for which he underwent aortography.

Box 3.1 Indications for thoracic and lumbar radiographs

- Major trauma
- Impaired consciousness
- Distracting injury
- Physical signs of thoracic or lumbar trauma
- Pelvic fractures
- Altered peripheral neurology

sustained (because of the frequency with which injuries at more than one level coexist) or if signs of thoracic or lumbar trauma are detected when the patient is log rolled. In obtunded patients in whom the thoracic and lumbar spine cannot be evaluated clinically, the radiographs should be obtained routinely during the secondary survey or on admission to hospital. Unstable fractures of the pelvis are often associated with injuries to the lumbar spine.

A significant force is normally required to damage the thoracic, lumbar, and sacral segments of the spinal cord, and the skeletal injury is usually evident on the standard anteroposterior and horizontal beam lateral radiographs. Burst fractures, and fractures affecting the posterior facet joints or pedicles, are unstable and more easily seen on the lateral radiograph. Instability requires at least two of the three columns of the spine to be disrupted. In simple wedge fractures, only the anterior column is disrupted and the injury remains stable. The demonstration of detail in the thoracic spine can be extremely difficult, particularly in the upper four vertebrae, and computed tomography (CT) is often required

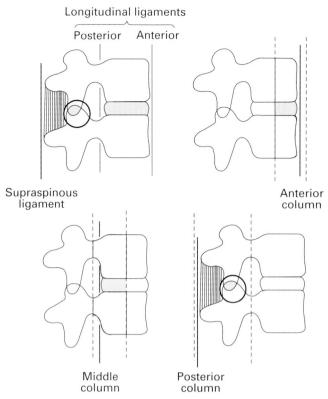

Figure 3.13 The three (anterior, middle and posterior) spinal columns. (Reproduced, with permission, from Denis F. *Spine* 1993;**8**:817–31).

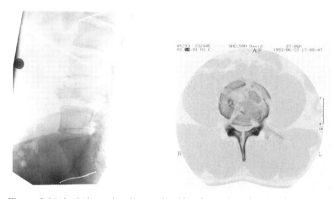

Figure 3.14 Left: lateral radiograph of lumbar spine showing burst fracture of L4 in a patient with a cauda equina lesion. Right: CT scan shows the fracture of L4 more clearly, with severe narrowing of the spinal canal.

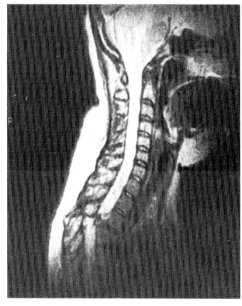

Figure 3.15 MRI showing transection of the spinal cord associated with a fracture of T4.

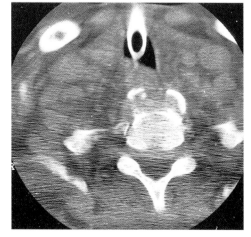

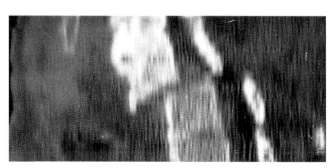

Figure 3.16 Left: CT scan with (right) sagittal reconstruction showing C7–T1 bilateral facet dislocation—a useful technique at the cervicothoracic junction.

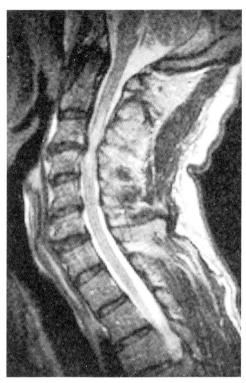

Figure 3.17 MRI showing C3–4 central disc prolapse with spinal cord compression and an area of high signal in the cord indicating oedema.

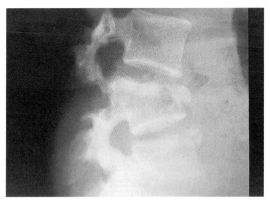

Figure 3.18 Chance fracture of L4 in a 17-year-old back-seat passenger, wearing a lap seat belt. There is a horizontal fracture of the upper part of the vertebral body extending into the posterior elements. There is also wedging of the body of L4 and more minor wedging of L5.

Further reading

- Brandser EA, el-Khoury GY. Thoracic and lumbar spine trauma. *Radiol Clin North Am* 1997;**35**:533–57
- Daffner RH, ed. *Imaging of vertebral trauma*. Philadelphia: Lippincott-Raven, 1996
- Hoffman JR, Mower WR, Wolfson AB *et al.* Validity of a set of clinical criteria to rule out injury to the cervical spine in patients with blunt trauma. *New Engl J Med* 2000;**343**:94–9
- Jones KE, Wakeley CJ, Jewell F. Another line of enquiry (atlanto-occipital dislocation). *Injury* 1995;**26**:195–8
- Kathol MH. Cervical spine trauma. What is new? *Radiol Clin North Am* 1997;**35**:507–32
- Nicholson DA, Driscoll PA, eds. *ABC of emergency radiology*. London: BMJ Publishing Group, 1995

for better definition. Instability in thoracic spinal injuries may also be caused by sternal or bilateral rib fractures, as the anterior splinting effect of these structures will be lost.

A particular type of fracture, the Chance fracture, is typically found in the upper lumbar vertebrae. It runs transversely through the vertebral body and usually results from a shearing force exerted by the lap component of a seat belt during severe deceleration injury. These fractures are often associated with intra-abdominal or retroperitoneal injuries.

A haematoma in the posterior mediastinum is often seen around the thoracic fracture site, particularly in the anteroposterior view of the spine and sometimes on the chest radiograph requested in the primary survey. If there is any suspicion that these appearances might be due to traumatic aortic dissection, an arch aortogram will be required.

Fractures in the thoracic and lumbar spine are often complex and inadequately shown on plain films. CT demonstrates bony detail more accurately. MRI is used to demonstrate the extent of cord and soft tissue damage.

4 Early management and complications—I

David Grundy, Andrew Swain

Respiratory complications

Respiratory insufficiency is common in patients with injuries of the cervical cord. If the neurological lesion is complete the patient will have paralysed intercostal muscles and will have to rely on diaphragmatic respiration. Partial paralysis of the diaphragm may also be present, either from the outset or after 24–48 hours if ascending post-traumatic cord oedema develops. In patients with injuries of the thoracic spine, respiratory impairment often results from associated rib fractures, haemopneumothorax, or pulmonary contusion; there may also be a varying degree of intercostal paralysis depending on the neurological level of the lesion.

Sputum retention occurs readily during the first few days after injury, particularly in patients with high lesions and in those with associated chest injury. The inability to produce an effective cough impairs the clearing of secretions and commonly leads to atelectasis. The loss of lung compliance contributes to difficulty in breathing and leads to a rapid exhaustion of the inspiratory muscles. Abnormal distribution of gases and blood (ventilation-perfusion mismatch) also occurs in the lungs of tetraplegic patients, producing further respiratory impairment.

Patients normally need to be nursed in the recumbent position because of the spinal injury, and even if spinal stabilisation has been undertaken, tetraplegics and high paraplegics should still not be sat up, as this position limits the excursion of the diaphragm and reduces their vital capacity.

Regular chest physiotherapy with assisted coughing and breathing exercises is vital to prevent atelectasis and pulmonary infection. Respiratory function should be monitored by measuring the oxygen saturation, vital capacity, and arterial blood gases. A vital capacity of less than 15 ml/kg body weight with a rising Pco_2 denotes respiratory failure, and should alert clinicians to support respiration (non-invasive pressure support may suffice). Bi-level support is preferable to continuous positive airway pressure (CPAP) and may avoid resorting to full ventilation. This mode of respiratory support may also assist in weaning the patient from full ventilation. The inspired air must be humified, as in full ventilation, otherwise secretions will become viscid and difficult to clear.

If atelectasis necessitates bronchoscopy this is a safe procedure which can be performed without undue movement of the patient's neck by using modern fibreoptic instruments. If the patient is already intubated the fibreoptic bronchoscope can be passed down the tracheal tube. Although early tracheostomy is best avoided in the first instance, as ventilation is sometimes needed for a few days only, it should not be delayed unnecessarily. It allows easy access for airways toilet and facilitates weaning from the ventilator. Minitracheostomy can be useful if the problem is purely one of retained secretions.

A patient whose respiratory function is initially satisfactory after injury but then deteriorates should regain satisfactory ventilatory capacity once spinal cord oedema subsides. Artificial ventilation should therefore not be withheld, except perhaps in the elderly and infirm where treatment is likely to be prolonged and unsuccessful. By involving the patients and their relatives, artificial ventilation may sometimes be withheld in this situation and the patient kept comfortable. If there is a risk of

---

Box 4.1 Causes of respiratory insufficiency

In tetraplegia:
Intercostal paralysis
Partial phrenic nerve palsy—immediate
　　　　　　　　　　　　　—delayed
Impaired ability to expectorate
Ventilation-perfusion mismatch

In paraplegia:
Variable intercostal paralysis according to level of injury
Associated chest injuries
—rib fractures
—pulmonary contusion
—haemopneumothorax

Box 4.2 Nurse in recumbent position to:

- Protect the spinal cord
- Maximise diaphragmatic excursion

Box 4.3 Physiotherapy

- Regular chest physiotherapy
- Assisted coughing

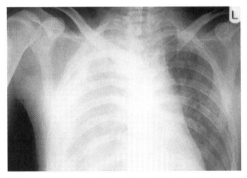

Figure 4.1 Chest radiograph on the day of injury in a 30 year old motorcyclist with a T6 fracture and paraplegia. There are bilateral haemothoraces, more severe on the right. Chest drains were required on both sides.

deterioration in respiratory function during transit, an anaesthetist must accompany the patient. Cardiac failure after spinal cord injury is often secondary to respiratory failure.

Weaning from pressure support or full ventilation should be managed with the patient in the recumbent position to take advantage of maximal diaphragmatic excursion.

With increasing public awareness of cardiopulmonary resuscitation and the routine attendance of paramedics at accidents, patients with high cervical injuries and complete phrenic nerve paralysis are surviving. These patients often require long-term ventilatory support, and this can be achieved either mechanically or electronically by phrenic nerve pacing in selected cases, although not all high tetraplegics are suitable for phrenic nerve pacing. If the spinal cord injury causes damage to the anterior horn cells of C3, C4 and C5, the phrenic nerve will have lower motor neurone damage and be incapable of being stimulated. The necessity for long-term ventilation should be no bar to the patient returning home, and patients are now surviving on domiciliary ventilation with a satisfactory quality of life (see Chapter 14).

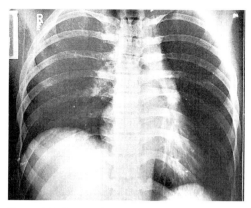

Figure 4.2 Chest radiograph: right diaphragmatic paralysis resulting from ascending cord oedema developing 48 hours after the patient had sustained complete tetraplegia below C4 because of C3–4 dislocation.

Cardiovascular complications

Haemorrhage from associated injuries is the commonest cause of post-traumatic shock and must be treated vigorously. However, it must be realised that in traumatic tetraplegia the thoracolumbar (T1–L2) sympathetic outflow is interrupted. Vagal tone is therefore unopposed and the patient can become hypotensive and bradycardic. Even in paraplegia, sympathetic paralysis below the lesion can produce hypotension, referred to as neurogenic shock. If shock is purely neurogenic in origin, patients can mistakenly be given large volumes of intravenous fluid and then develop pulmonary oedema.

Pharyngeal suction and tracheal intubation stimulate the vagus, and in high cord injuries can produce bradycardia, which may result in cardiac arrest. To prevent this it is wise to give atropine or glycopyrronium in addition to oxygen before suction and intubation are undertaken and also whenever the heart rate falls below 50 beats/minute. Clinicians, however, must be aware of the possible toxic effects when the standard dose of 0.6 mg atropine is used repeatedly. If the systolic blood pressure cannot maintain adequate perfusion pressure to produce an acceptable flow of urine after any hypovolaemia has been corrected, then inotropic medication with dopamine should be started.

Cardiac arrest due to sudden hyperkalaemia after the use of a depolarising agent such as suxamethonium for tracheal intubation is a risk in patients with spinal cord trauma between three days and nine months after injury. If muscle relaxation is required for intubation during this period a non-depolarising muscle relaxant such as rocuronium is indicated to avoid the risk of hyperkalaemic cardiac arrest.

Prophylaxis against thromboembolism

Newly injured tetraplegic or paraplegic patients have a very high risk of developing thromboembolic complications. The incidence of pulmonary embolism reaches a maximum in the third week after injury and it is the commonest cause of death in patients who survive the period immediately after the injury.

If there are no other injuries or medical contraindications, such as head or chest injury, antiembolism stockings should be applied to all patients and anticoagulation started within the

Box 4.4 Improved cardiopulmonary resuscitation

- Increased number of high lesion tetraplegics now survive the acute injury
- Many require long-term ventilatory support

Beware of overinfusion in patients with neurogenic shock

Treat
Bradycardia <50 beats/min
Hypotension <80 mm Hg systolic or adequate urinary excretion not maintained

Risk of hyperkalaemic cardiac arrest

Beware—*do not* give suxamethonium from three days to nine months following spinal cord injury as grave risk of hyperkalaemic cardiac arrest

Box 4.5 Anticoagulation

- Apply antiembolism stockings
- If there are no medical or surgical contraindications give low molecular weight heparin within 72 hours

first 72 hours of the accident. Low molecular weight heparin for 8–12 weeks is usually preferred to warfarin.

Initial bladder management

After a severe spinal cord injury the bladder is initially acontractile, and untreated the patient will develop acute retention. The volume of urine in the bladder should never be allowed to exceed 500 ml because overstretching the detrusor muscle can delay the return of bladder function. If the patient is transferred to a spinal injuries unit within a few hours after injury it may be possible to defer catheterisation until then, but if the patient drank a large volume of fluid before injury this is unwise. In these circumstances, and in patients with multiple injuries, the safest course is to pass a small bore (12–14 Ch) 10 ml balloon silicone Foley catheter.

The gastrointestinal tract

The patient should receive intravenous fluids for at least the first 48 hours, as paralytic ileus usually accompanies a severe spinal injury. A nasogastric tube is passed and oral fluids are forbidden until normal bowel sounds return. If paralytic ileus becomes prolonged the abdominal distension splints the diaphragm and, particularly in tetraplegic patients, this may precipitate a respiratory crisis if not relieved by nasogastric aspiration. If a tetraplegic patient vomits, gastric contents are easily aspirated because the patient cannot cough effectively. Ileus may also be precipitated by an excessive lumbar lordosis if too bulky a lumbar pillow is used for thoracolumbar injuries.

Acute peptic ulceration, with haemorrhage or perforation, is an uncommon but dangerous complication after spinal cord injury, and for this reason proton pump inhibitors or H_2-receptor antagonists should be started as soon as possible after injury and continued for at least three weeks. When perforation occurs it often presents a week after injury with referred pain to the shoulder, but during the stage of spinal shock guarding and rigidity will be absent and tachycardia may not develop. A supine decubitus abdominal film usually shows free gas in the peritoneal cavity.

Use of steroids and antibiotics

An American study (NASCIS 2) suggested that a short course of high-dose methylprednisolone started within the first eight hours after closed spinal cord injury improves neurological outcome. A later study (NASCIS 3) suggested that patients commencing methylprednisolone within 3 hours of injury should have a 24-hour treatment regimen, but for patients commencing treatment 3–8 hours after injury the treatment period should be extended to 48 hours. Recently the use of steroids has been challenged, and their use has not been universally accepted. Policy concerning steroid treatment should be agreed with the local spinal injuries unit.

Antibiotics are not normally indicated for the prevention of either urinary or pulmonary infection. Only established infections should be treated.

The skin and pressure areas

When the patient is transferred from trolley to bed the whole of the back must be inspected for bruising, abrasions, or signs of pressure on the skin. The patient should be turned every two

---

Box 4.6 Initial bladder management

- Avoid overdistension
- 12–14 Ch silicone Foley catheter

Beware of paralytic ileus: patients should receive intravenous fluids for at least the first 48 hours after injury

---

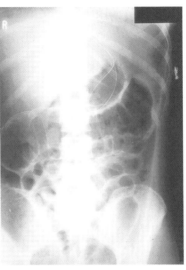

(a)

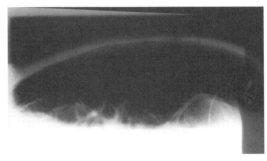

(b)

Figure 4.3 a) Supine abdominal x ray demonstrating the double lumen sign (gas inside and outside the bowel) in an acute perforated gastric ulcer occurring in a tetraplegic 5 days post-injury. b) Supine decubitus view showing massive collection of free gas under the anterior abdominal wall.

Box 4.7 Risk of acute peptic ulceration with haemorrhage or perforation

- Treat with proton pump inhibitor or H_2-receptor antagonist
- Continue treatment for three weeks

Box 4.8 Drug treatment in spinal cord injury

- Consult your spinal unit for advice
- If methylprednisolone is given, administer at the earliest opportunity: 30 mg/kg intravenously and then infusion of 5.4 mg/kg/h for 23 hours if commenced within 3 hours of injury. If treatment is started 3–8 hours after injury, the infusion is continued for 47 hours.

hours between supine and right and left lateral positions to prevent pressure sores, and the skin should be inspected at each turn. Manual turning can be achieved on a standard hospital bed, by lifting patients to one side (using the method described in chapter 8 on nursing) and then log rolling them into the lateral position. Alternatively, an electrically driven turning and tilting bed can be used. Another convenient solution is the Stryker frame, in which a patient is "sandwiched" between anterior and posterior sections, which can then be turned between the supine and prone positions by the inbuilt circular turning mechanism, but tetraplegic patients may not tolerate the prone position.

Nursing care requires the use of pillows to separate the legs, maintain alignment of the spine, and prevent the formation of contractures. In injuries of the cervical spine a neck roll is used to maintain cervical lordosis. A lumbar pillow maintains lumbar lordosis in thoracolumbar injuries.

Care of the joints and limbs

The joints must be passively moved through the full range each day to prevent stiffness and contractures in those joints which may later recover function and to prevent contractures elsewhere, which might interfere with rehabilitation. Splints to keep the tetraplegic hand in the position of function are particularly important. Foot drop and equinus contracture are prevented by placing a vertical pillow between the foot of the bed and the soles of the feet.

Skeletal traction of lower limb fractures should be avoided, but early internal or external fixation of limb fractures is often indicated to assist nursing, particularly as pressure sores in anaesthetic areas may develop unnoticed in plaster casts.

Later analgesia

In the ward environment, diamorphine administered as a low-dose subcutaneous constant infusion, once the correct initial dose has been titrated, gives excellent pain relief, especially if combined with a non-steroidal anti-inflammatory drug. Close observation is essential and naloxone must always be available in case of respiratory depression.

It diamorphine is unavailable, a syringe-driven intraveneous morphine infusion can be used.

Trauma re-evaluation

Trauma patients may be obtunded by head injury or distracted by major fractures and wounds. As a result, some injuries associated with high morbidity, for example scaphoid fracture, may not generate symptoms during early management. The diagnosis of such injuries can be difficult in any trauma patient but in spinal cord injury, the symptoms and signs are often abolished by sensory and motor impairments. Furthermore, some of these injuries compromise rehabilitation and the ultimate functional outcome. Daily re-evaluation of trauma patients helps to overcome these diagnostic difficulties and is very important during the first month after injury.

Further reading

- Bracken MB *et al.* Administration of methylprednisolone for 24 or 48 hours or tirilazad mesylate for 48 hours in the treatment of acute spinal cord injury. *JAMA* 1997;**277**:1597–604

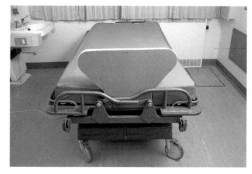

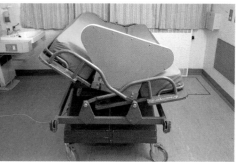

Figure 4.4 Electrically-powered turning and tilting bed in (upper) supine position and (lower) left lateral position. In the lateral position, note the slight tilt on the opposing side to prevent the patient sliding out of alignment.

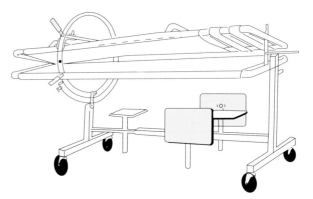

Figure 4.5 Stryker frame.

Box 4.9 Joint and limb care

- Daily passive movement of joints
- Splints for hands of tetraplegic patients
- Early internal fixation of limb fractures often required

Box 4.10 Trauma re-evaluation

Following spinal cord trauma, occult injuries can easily compromise recovery or aggravate disability. Complete clinical re-assessments must be performed regularly during the first month after injury

- Chen CF, Lien IN, Wu MC. Respiratory function in patients with spinal cord injuries: effects of posture. *Paraplegia* 1990;**28**:81–6
- Menter RR, Bach J, Brown DJ, Gutteridge G, Watt J. A review of the respiratory management of a patient with high level tetraplegia. *Spinal Cord* 1997;**35**:805–8
- Short DJ, El Masry WS, Jones PW. High dose methylprednisolone in the management of acute spinal cord injury—a systematic review from a clinical perspective. *Spinal Cord* 2000;**38**:273–86
- Tromans AM, Mecci M, Barrett FH, Ward TA, Grundy DJ. The use of BiPAP biphasic positive airway pressure system in acute spinal cord injury. *Spinal Cord* 1998;**36**:481–4

5 Early management and complications—II

David Grundy, Andrew Swain

The anatomy of spinal cord injury

The radiographic appearances of the spine after injury are not a reliable guide to the severity of spinal cord damage. They represent the final or "recoil" position of the vertebrae and do not necessarily indicate the forces generated in the injury. The spinal cord ends at the lower border of the first lumbar vertebra in adults, the remainder of the spinal canal being occupied by the nerve roots of the cauda equina. There is greater room for the neural structures in the cervical and lumbar canals, but in the thoracic region the spinal cord diameter and that of the neural canal more nearly approximate. The blood supply of the cervical spinal cord is good, whereas that of the thoracic cord, especially at its midpoint, is relatively poor. These factors may explain the greater preponderance of complete lesions seen after injuries to the thoracic spine. The initial injury is mechanical, but there is usually an early ischaemic lesion that may rapidly progress to cord necrosis. Extension of this, often many segments below the level of the lesion, accounts for the observation that on occasion patients have lower motor neurone or flaccid paralysis when upper motor neurone or spastic paralysis would have been expected from the site of the bony injury. Because of the potential for regeneration of peripheral nerves, neurological recovery is unpredictable in lesions of the cauda equina.

The spinal injury

Treatment should be aimed at stabilising the spine to avoid further damage by movement and also to relieve cord compression.

The cervical spine

Patients with injuries of the cervical spine should initially be managed by skeletal traction. Applied through skull calipers, traction is aimed at reducing any fracture or dislocation, relieving pressure on the cord in the case of burst fractures, and splinting the spine.

Of the various skull calipers available, spring-loaded types such as the Gardner-Wells are the most suitable for inserting in the emergency department. Local anaesthetic is infiltrated into the scalp down to the periosteum about 2.5 cm above the pinna at the site of the maximum bitemporal diameter, and the caliper is then screwed into the scalp to grip the outer table of the skull. No incisions need be made, and the spring loading of one of the screws determines when the correct tension has been reached. The University of Virginia caliper is similar in action and easily applied. The Cone caliper is satisfactory but requires small scalp incisions and the drilling of 1 mm impressions in the outer table of the skull. Insertion too far anteriorly interferes with temporalis function and causes trismus. The Crutchfield caliper is no longer recommended because of the high incidence of complications.

When the upper cervical spine is injured less traction is required for reduction and stabilisation. Usually 1–2 kg is enough for stabilisation; if more weight is used overdistraction at the site of injury may cause neurological deterioration. Specific injuries of the upper cervical spine and the cervicothoracic junction are discussed in chapter 6.

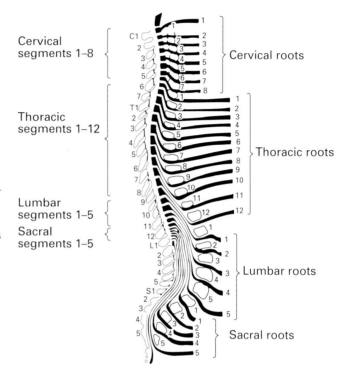

Cervical segments 1–8

Thoracic segments 1–12

Lumbar segments 1–5

Sacral segments 1–5

Cervical roots

Thoracic roots

Lumbar roots

Sacral roots

Figure 5.1 Anatomy of spinal cord injury.

Box 5.1 Skull traction used

- To reduce dislocation
- To relieve pressure on spinal cord in case of burst fractures
- To splint the spine

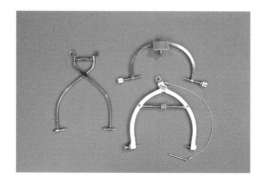

Figure 5.2 Cone (left), Gardner-Wells (upper right), and University of Virginia (lower right) calipers.

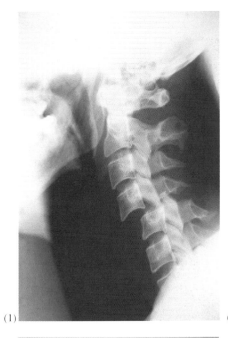
(1)

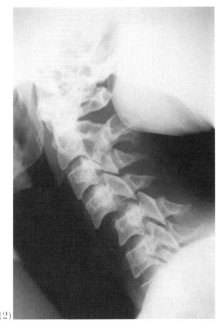
(2)

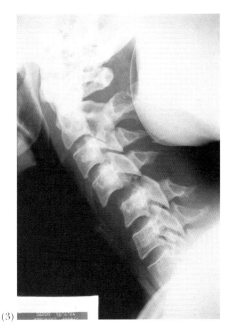
(3)

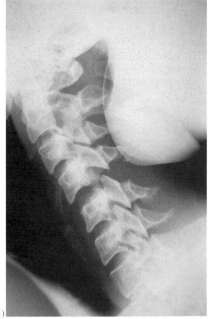
(4)

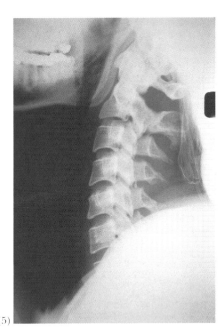
(5)

Figure 5.3 Reduction of a C4–5 bilateral facet dislocation due to severe flexion injury. Increasing traction weight was applied with the neck in flexion for 3.5 hours to 25 kg ((1)–(4)). (5) shows the final position after 4 hours with head extended and weight reduced to 4 kg traction. The neurological level improved from C5 to C6.

A traction force of 3–5 kg is normally applied to the calipers in fractures of the lower cervical spine without dislocation. A neck roll (not a sandbag) should be placed behind the neck to maintain the normal cervical lordosis. Pressure sores of the scalp in the occipital region are common, and care must be taken to cushion the occiput when positioning the patient. When necessary this can be achieved by using a suitably covered fluid-filled plastic bag, having ensured that there is no matted hair that could act as a source of pressure. If the spine is dislocated reduction can usually be achieved by increasing the weight by about 4 kg every 30 minutes (sometimes up to a total of 25 kg) with the neck in flexion until the facets are disengaged. The neck is then extended and the traction decreased to maintenance weight. The patient must be examined neurologically before each increment, and the traction force must be reduced immediately if the neurology deteriorates.

Manipulation under general anaesthesia is an alternative method of reduction, but, although complete neurological recovery has been reported after this procedure, there have been adverse effects in some patients and manipulation should

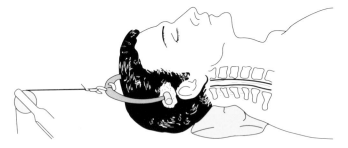

Figure 5.4 Skull traction using Gardner-Wells caliper, with neck roll in position.

only be attempted by specialists. Use of an image intensifier may facilitate such reductions.

Halo traction is a useful alternative to skull calipers, particularly in patients with incomplete tetraplegia, and conversion to a halo brace permits early mobilisation.

Skull traction is a satisfactory treatment for unstable injuries of the cervical spine in the early stages, but when the spinal cord lesion is incomplete, early operative fusion may be indicated to prevent further neurological damage. The decision to operate may sometimes be made before the patient is transferred to the spinal injuries unit, and if so the spinal unit should be consulted and management planned jointly.

Another indication for operation is an open wound, such as that following a gunshot or stab injury. Exploration or debridement should be performed.

Skull traction is unnecessary for patients with cervical spondylosis who sustain a hyperextension injury with tetraplegia but have no fracture or dislocation. In these circumstances the patient should be nursed with the head in slight flexion but otherwise free from restriction.

The thoracic and lumbar spine

Most thoracic and lumbar injuries are caused by flexion-rotation forces. Conservative treatment for injuries associated with cord damage is designed to minimise spinal movement, and to support the patient to maintain the correct posture. In practice a pillow under the lumbar spine to preserve normal lordosis is sometimes used. Dislocations of the thoracic and lumbar spine may sometimes be reduced by this technique of "postural reduction". However, internal fixation is recommended in some patients with unstable fracture-dislocations to prevent further cord or nerve root damage, correct deformity, and facilitate nursing. As yet there is no convincing evidence that internal fixation aids neurological recovery.

Transfer to a spinal injuries unit

In the United Kingdom, there are only 11 spinal injuries units and most patients will be admitted to a district general hospital for their initial treatment. As soon as spinal cord injury is diagnosed or suspected the nearest spinal injuries unit should be contacted. Immediate transfer is ideal, as management in an acute specialised unit is associated with reduced mortality, increased neurological recovery, shorter length of stay and reduced cost of care, compared to treatment in a non-specialised centre. The objects of management are to prevent further spinal cord damage by appropriate reduction and stabilisation of the spine, to prevent secondary neuronal injury, and to prevent medical complications.

The choice between immediate or early transfer will depend on the general condition of the patient and also on the intensive care facilities available. Unfortunately, some patients will not be fit enough for immediate transfer because of multiple injuries or severe respiratory impairment. In such cases it is advisable to consult, and perhaps arrange a visit by, a spinal injuries consultant. Transfer to a spinal injuries centre is most easily accomplished by means of a Stryker frame, which can be fitted with a constant tension device for skull traction. The RAF pattern turning frame is similarly equipped and was specifically developed for use by the Royal Air Force. In civilian practice, studies have shown that patients can be safely transferred from emergency departments using the standard

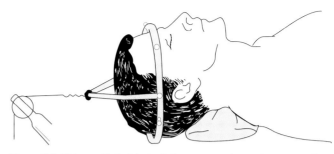

Figure 5.5 Halo applied with the bale arm—an alternative approach to skull traction if early mobilisation into a halo brace is being considered.

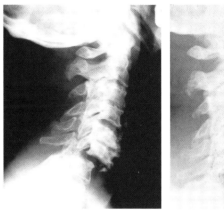 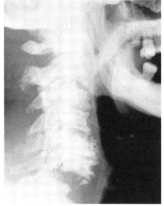

Figure 5.6 Left: bilateral facet dislocation in a patient with associated cervical spondylosis. Right: incorrect traction—too great a weight and head in extension—leading to distraction with neurological deterioration.

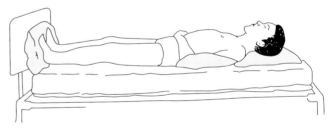

Figure 5.7 Support position for nursing a patient with a thoracolumbar spinal injury.

Box 5.2 Objects of early transfer to a spinal injuries unit

- To prevent further spinal cord damage by reduction and stabilisation of spine
- To prevent secondary neuronal injury
- To prevent medical complications
- To expedite all aspects of rehabilitation

Box 5.3 Delay in transfer to spinal injuries unit if:

Patient unfit to transfer—multiple injuries
        —need for emergency surgery
        —severe respiratory impairment
        —cardiorespiratory instability
Consider visit by spinal injuries consultant

techniques for cervical immobilisation described earlier. Tetraplegic patients should be accompanied by a suitably experienced doctor with anaesthetic skills, who can quickly intubate the patient if respiratory difficulty ensues. Transfer by helicopter is often the ideal and is advisable if the patient has to travel a long distance.

Further reading

- Grundy DJ. Skull traction and its complications. *Injury* 1983;**15**:173–7
- Mumford J, Weinstein JN, Spratt KF, Goel VK. Thoracolumbar burst fractures. The clinical efficacy and outcome of nonoperative management. *Spine* 1993; **18**:955–70
- Tator CH, Duncan EG, Edmonds VE, Lapczak LI, Andrews DF. Neurological recovery, mortality and length of stay after acute spinal cord injury associated with changes in management. *Paraplegia* 1995;**33**:254–62
- Vinken PJ, Bruyn GW, Klawans HL, eds. *Handbook of clinical neurology. Revised series 17. Spinal cord trauma*, vol 61 (co-edited by Frankel HL). Amsterdam: Elsevier Science Publishers, 1992

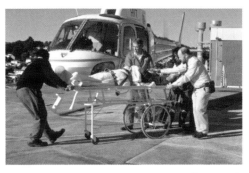

Figure 5.8 Helicopter transfer of a spinally injured patient.

6   Medical management in the spinal injuries unit

David Grundy, Anthony Tromans, John Carvell, Firas Jamil

Management of spinal cord injury in an acute specialised unit is associated with reduced mortality, increased neurological recovery, shorter length of stay and reduced cost of care, compared to treatment in a non-specialised centre. The objects of management are to prevent further spinal cord damage by appropriate reduction and stabilisation of the spine, to prevent secondary neuronal injury, and to prevent medical complications.

> **Box 6.1 Objectives of medical management**
>
> - Prevent further damage through reduction and immobilisation
> - Prevent secondary neuronal injury
> - Prevent medical complications

The cervical spine

In injuries of the cervical spine skull traction is normally maintained for six weeks initially. The spine may be positioned in neutral or extension depending on the nature of the injury. Thus flexion injuries with suspected or obvious damage to the posterior ligamentous complex are treated by placing the neck in a degree of extension. The standard site of insertion of skull calipers need not be changed to achieve this; extension is achieved by correctly positioning a pillow or support under the shoulders. Most injuries are managed with the neck in the neutral position. An appropriately sized neck roll can also be inserted to maintain normal cervical lordosis and for the comfort of the patient.

The application of a halo brace is a useful alternative to skull traction in many patients, once the neck is reduced. It provides stability and allows early mobilisation. Its use is often necessary for up to 12 weeks, when it can be replaced by a cervical collar if the neck is stable.

One of the most difficult aspects of cervical spine injury management is assessment of stability. Radiographs are taken regularly for position and at six weeks for evidence of bony union, immobilisation being continued for a further two to

> **Box 6.2 Cervical spine injuries**
>
> - Skull traction for at least six weeks
> - Halo traction—allows early mobilisation by conversion into halo brace in selected patients
> - Spinal fusion —acute central disc prolapse (urgent decompression required)
>   —severe ligamentous damage
>   —correction of major spinal deformity

> **Box 6.3 Radiological signs of instability seen on standard lateral radiographs or flexion-extension views**
>
> - Widening of gap between adjacent spinous processes
> - Widening of intervertebral disc space
> - Greater than 3.5 mm anterior or posterior displacement of vertebral body
> - Increased angulation between adjacent vertebrae

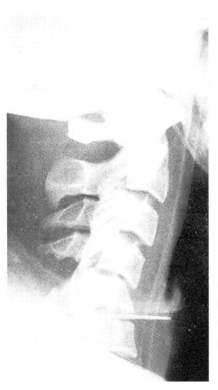
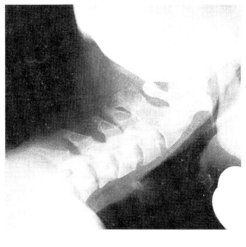
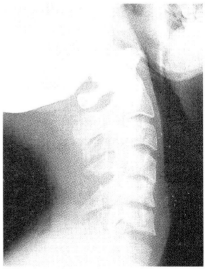

Figure 6.1 Left: unstable flexion injury in a man who sustained complete tetraplegia below C5. Note forward slip of C4 on C5 and widened interspinous gap, indicating posterior ligament damage. Middle and right: same patient six months later conservatively treated. Flexion-extension views show no appreciable movement but a persisting slight flexion deformity at the site of the previous instability.

three weeks if there are any signs of instability. Once stability is achieved the patient is sat up in bed gradually during the course of a few days, wearing a firm cervical support such as a Philadelphia or Miami collar, before being mobilised into a wheelchair. This process is most conveniently achieved with a profiling bed, but the skin over the natal cleft and other pressure areas must be inspected frequently for signs of pressure or shearing. Some patients, particularly those with high level lesions, have postural hypotension when first mobilised because of their sympathetic paralysis, so profiling must not be hurried.

Antiembolism stockings and an abdominal binder help reduce the peripheral pooling of blood due to the sympathetic paralysis. Ephedrine 15–30 mg given 20 minutes before profiling starts is also effective. Once the spine is radiologically stable the firm collar can often be dispensed with at about 12 weeks after injury and a soft collar worn for comfort.

Twelve weeks after injury following plain *x* ray, if there is any likelihood of instability, flexion-extension radiography should be performed under medical supervision but if pain or paraesthesiae occur the procedure must be discontinued. It must be remembered that pain-induced muscle spasm may mask ligamentous injury and give a false sense of security. Most unstable injuries in the lower cervical spine are due to flexion or flexion-rotation forces and in the upper cervical spine to hyperextension. If internal fixation is indicated an anterior or posterior approach can be used, but if there is anterior cord compression, such as by a disc, anterior decompression and fixation is necessary. Fixation must be sound to avoid the need for extensive additional support.

The decision to perform spinal fusion is usually taken early, and sometimes it will have been performed in the district general hospital before transfer to the spinal injuries unit. The decision about when to operate will depend on the expertise and facilities available and the condition of the patient, but we suspect from our experience that early surgery in high lesion patients can sometimes precipitate respiratory failure, requiring prolonged ventilation. Some patients require late spinal fusion because of failed conservative treatment.

The upper cervical spine

As injuries of the upper cervical spine are often initially associated with acute respiratory failure, prompt appropriate treatment is important, including ventilation if necessary. Other patients may have little or no neurological deficit but again prompt treatment is important to prevent neurological deterioration.

Fractures of the atlas are of two types. The most common, a fracture of the posterior arch, is due to an extension-compression force and is a stable injury which can be safely treated by immobilisation in a firm collar. The second type, the Jefferson fracture, is due to a vertical compression force to the vertex of the skull, resulting in the occipital condyles being driven downwards to produce a bursting injury, in which there is outward displacement of the lateral masses of the atlas and in which the transverse ligament may also have been ruptured. This is an unstable injury with the potential for atlanto-axial instability, and skull traction or immobilisation in a halo brace is necessary for at least eight weeks.

Fractures through the base of the odontoid process (type II fractures) are usually caused by hyperextension, and result in posterior displacement of the odontoid and posterior subluxation of C1 on C2; flexion injuries produce anterior displacement of the odontoid and anterior subluxation of C1 on C2. If displacement is considerable, reduction is achieved

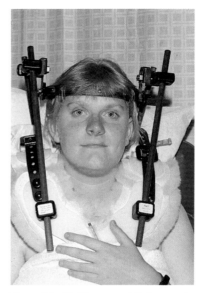

Figure 6.2 C2 ("hangman's") fracture immobilised and treated in a halo brace compatible with the use of CT and MRI.

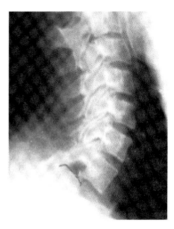
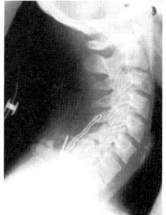

Figure 6.3 C7–T1 bilateral facet dislocation with fractures of spinous processes of C6 and C7 and complete tetraplegia below C7. Treated by operative reduction and stabilisation by wiring the spinous processes of C5 to T1 and bone grafting.

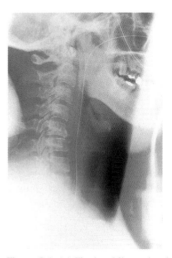
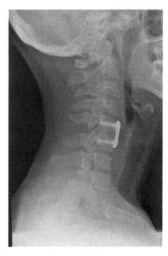

Figure 6.4 (a) Flexion/distraction injury in a 42-year-old female, with a Brown–Séquard syndrome. Note the fanning of the spinous processes of C5 and C6, angulation between the bodies of C5 and C6, and bony fragments anteriorly. MRI showed central disc prolapse at C5-6 with cord compression. (b) She underwent a C5-6 anterior cervical discectomy, bone grafting and anterior cervical plating. She made an almost complete neurological recovery.

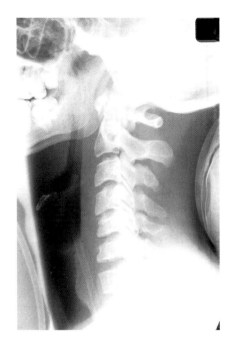

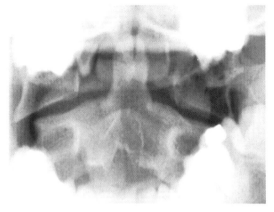

Figure 6.5 Left: lateral view of diving injury with compression fractures of the bodies of C5 and C6 and an associated Jefferson fracture of the atlas not obvious on this view. Right: anteroposterior view shows Jefferson fracture clearly with outward displacement of the right lateral mass of the atlas.

by gentle controlled skull traction under radiographic control. Immobilisation is continued for at least three to four months, depending on radiographic signs of healing. Halo bracing is very useful in managing this fracture. Atlanto-axial fusion may be undertaken by the anterior or posterior route if there is non-union and atlanto-axial instability. Anterior odontoid screw fixation may prevent rotational instability and avoid the need for a halo brace.

The "hangman's" fracture, a traumatic spondylolisthesis of the axis, so called because the bony damage is similar to that seen in judicial hanging, is usually produced by hyperextension of the head on the neck, or less commonly with flexion. This results in a fracture through the pedicles of the axis in the region of the pars interarticularis, with an anterior slip of the C2 vertebral body on that of C3. Bony union occurs readily, but gentle skull traction should be maintained for six weeks, followed by immobilisation in a firm collar for a further two months. Great care must be taken to avoid overdistraction in this injury. Indeed, in all upper cervical fracture-dislocations once reduction has been achieved control can usually be obtained by reducing the traction force to only 1–2 kg. If more weight is used, neurological deterioration may result from overdistraction at the site of injury. An alternative approach when there is no bony displacement or when reduction has been achieved is to apply a halo brace. This avoids overdistraction from skull traction.

Ankylosing spondylitis predisposes the spine to fracture. It must be remembered that in this condition the neck is normally flexed, and to straighten the cervical spine will tend to cause respiratory obstruction, increase the deformity and risk further spinal cord damage. Help should be sought as soon as the problem is recognised.

The cervicothoracic junction

Closed reduction of a C7–T1 facet dislocation is often difficult if not impossible, in which case operative reduction by facetectomy and posterior fusion is indicated, particularly in patients with an incomplete spinal cord lesion.

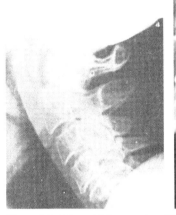
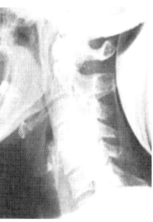

Figure 6.6 Odontoid fracture in a 64-year-old woman due to hyperextension injury after a fall on to her face at home. It was reduced by applying 4 kg traction force, with atlanto-occipital flexion; the position was subsequently maintained by using a reduced weight of 1.5 kg.

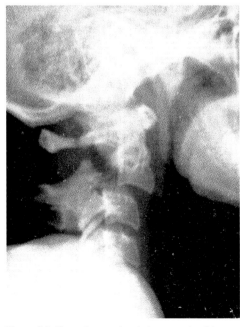

Figure 6.7 Forced extension injury sustained in a car accident by a 22-year-old woman, resulting in "hangman's" fracture. There is also associated fracture of the posterior arch of the atlas.

Thoracic injuries

The anatomy of the thoracic spine and the rib cage gives it added stability, although injuries to the upper thoracic spine are sometimes associated with a fracture of the sternum, which makes the injury unstable because of the loss of the normal anterior splinting effect of the sternum. It is very difficult to brace the upper thoracic spine, and if such a patient is mobilised too quickly a severe flexion deformity of the spine may develop.

In the majority of patients with a thoracic spinal cord injury, the neurological deficit is complete, and patients are usually managed conservatively by six to eight weeks' bed rest.

Thoracolumbar and lumbar injuries

Most patients with thoracolumbar injuries can be managed conservatively with an initial period of bed rest for 8 to 12 weeks followed by gradual mobilisation in a spinal brace. If there is gross deformity or if the injury is unstable, especially if the spinal cord injury is incomplete, operative reduction, surgical instrumentation, and bone grafting correct the deformity and permit early mobilisation.

Isolated laminectomy has no place because it may render the spine unstable and does not achieve adequate decompression of the spinal cord except in the rare instance of a depressed fracture of a lamina. It must be combined with internal fixation and bone grafting. If spinal cord decompression is felt to be desirable, surgery should be aimed at the site of bony compression, which is generally anteriorly. An anterior approach with vertebrectomy by an experienced surgeon carries little added morbidity, except that it may cause significant deterioration in patients with pulmonary or chest wall injury. Dislocations and translocations can be dealt with by a posterior approach.

Before a patient with an unstable injury is mobilised, the spine is braced, the brace remaining in place until bony union occurs. Even if operative reduction has been undertaken, bracing may still be required for up to six months, depending on the type of spinal fusion performed.

Deep vein thrombosis and pulmonary embolism

Due to the very high incidence of thromboembolic complications, prophylaxis using antiembolism stockings and low molecular weight heparin should, in the absence of contraindications, be started within the first 72 hours of the accident. It is continued throughout the initial period of bed rest until the patient is fully mobile in a wheelchair and for a total of 8 weeks, or 12 weeks if there are additional risk factors such as a history of deep vein thrombosis, a lower limb fracture, or obesity.

An alternative is to commence warfarin as soon as the patient's paralytic ileus has settled. If pulmonary embolism occurs the management is as for non-paralysed patients.

Autonomic dysreflexia

Autonomic dysreflexia is seen particularly in patients with cervical cord injuries above the sympathetic outflow but may also occur in those with high thoracic lesions above T6. It may occur at any time after the period of spinal shock and is usually

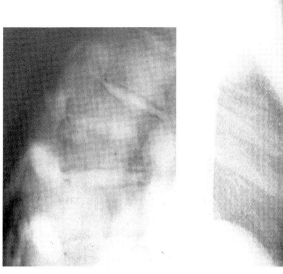

Figure 6.8 Wedge compression fractures of T5 and T6 in association with a fracture of the sternum.

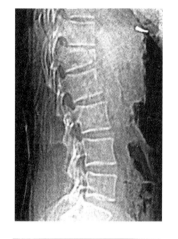
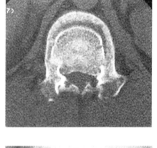
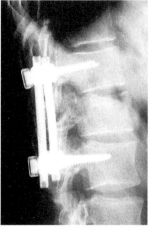
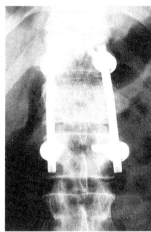

Figure 6.9 Lateral CT (scanogram) showing wedge compression fracture of L1 with incomplete paraplegia; axial view on CT showing canal encroachment and pedicular widening; after transpedicular fixation with restoration of vertebral height and alignment.

due to a distended bladder caused by a blocked catheter, or to poor bladder emptying as a result of detrusor-sphincter dyssynergia. The distension of the bladder results in reflex sympathetic overactivity below the level of the spinal cord lesion, causing vasoconstriction and severe systemic hypertension. The carotid and aortic baroreceptors are stimulated and respond via the vasomotor centre with increased vagal tone and resulting bradycardia, but the peripheral vasodilatation that would normally have relieved the hypertension does not occur because stimuli cannot pass distally through the injured cord.

Characteristically the patient suffers a pounding headache, profuse sweating, and flushing or blotchiness of the skin above the level of the spinal cord lesion. Without prompt treatment, intracranial haemorrhage may occur.

Other conditions in which visceral stimulation can result in autonomic dysreflexia include urinary tract infection, bladder calculi, a loaded colon, an anal fissure, ejaculation during sexual intercourse, and labour.

Treatment consists of removing the precipitating cause. If this lies in the urinary tract catheterisation is often necessary. If hypertension persists nifedipine 5–10 mg sublingually, glyceryl trinitrate 300 micrograms sublingually, or phentolamine 5–10 mg intravenously is given. If inadequately treated the patient can become sensitised and develop repeated attacks with minimal stimuli. Occasionally the sympathetic reflex activity may have to be blocked by a spinal or epidural anaesthetic. Later management may include removal of bladder calculi or sphincterotomy if detrusor-sphincter dyssynergia is causing the symptoms; performed under spinal anaesthesia, the risk of autonomic dysreflexia is lessened.

Biochemical disturbances

Hyponatraemia

The aetiology of hyponatraemia is multifactorial, involving fluid overload, diuretic usage, the sodium depleting effects of drugs such as carbamazepine, and inappropriate antidiuretic hormone secretion.

It may occur (1) during the acute stage of spinal cord injury, when the patient is on intravenous fluids, or (2) in the chronic phase, often in association with systemic sepsis frequently of chest or urinary tract origin, and often exacerbated by the patient increasing their oral fluid intake in an attempt to eradicate a suspected urinary infection.

Treatment depends on the severity and the cause. Sepsis should be controlled, fluids restricted, and medication reviewed. Hypertonic saline (2N) should be avoided because of the risk of central pontine myelinolysis. Furosemide (frusemide) and potassium supplements are useful, but the rate of correction of the serum sodium must be managed carefully.

Occasionally hyponatraemia is prolonged and in this situation demeclocycline hydrochloride is useful.

Hypercalcaemia

Any prolonged period of immobility results in the mobilisation of calcium from the bones, and, particularly in tetraplegics, this can be associated with symptomatic hypercalcaemia. The diagnosis is often difficult, and symptoms can include constipation, abdominal pain, and headaches. The problem is uncommon and diagnosis may be delayed, if the serum calcium is not measured.

Box 6.4 Autonomic dysreflexia

- Pounding headache
- Profuse sweating
- Flushing or blotchiness above level of lesion
- Danger of intracranial haemorrhage

Box 6.5 Treatment of autonomic dysreflexia

- Remove the cause
- Sit patient up
- Treat with:
    Nifedipine 5–10 mg capsule—bite and swallow
    or
    Glyceryl trinitrate 300 µg sublingually

If blood pressure continues to rise despite intervention, treat with antihypertensive drug e.g. phentolamine 5–10 mg intravenously in 2·5 mg increments

- Spinal or epidural anaesthetic (rarely)

Box 6.6 Biochemical disturbances

Hyponatraemia
Acute —due to excessive intravenous fluids
Chronic —systemic sepsis
—excessive oral fluid intake
—drug induced e.g. carbamazepine
Treatment—treat sepsis
—control fluid intake
—review drugs
—furosemide, potassium supplements
—demeclocycline (occasionally)

Hypercalcaemia
Symptoms—constipation
Treatment—hydration
—achieve diuresis
—oral disodium etidronate or intravenous disodium pamidronate

Treatment involves hydration, achieving a diuresis (with a fluid load and furosemide (frusemide)), and the use of oral sodium etidronate or intravenous disodium pamidronate. Once the patient is fully mobile the problem usually resolves.

Para-articular heterotopic ossification

After injury to the spinal cord new bone is often laid down in the soft tissues around paralysed joints, particularly the hip and knee. The cause is unknown, although local trauma has been suggested. It usually presents with erythema, induration, or swelling near a joint. There is pronounced osteoblastic activity, but the new bone formed does not mature for at least 18 months. This has an important bearing on treatment in that if excision of heterotopic bone is required because of gross restriction of movement or bony ankylosis of a joint, surgery is best delayed for at least 18 months—until the new bone is mature. Earlier surgical intervention may provoke further new bone formation, thus compounding the original condition. Treatment with disodium etidronate suppresses the mineralisation of osteoid tissue and may reverse up to half of early lesions when used for 3–6 months, and non-steroidal anti-inflammatory drugs are also used to prevent the progression of this complication. Postoperative radiotherapy may halt the recurrence of the problem if early surgical intervention has to be performed.

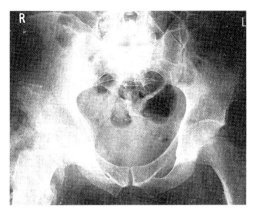

Figure 6.10 Heterotopic ossification in the right hip.

Spasticity

Spasticity is seen only in patients with upper motor neurone lesions of the cord whose intact spinal reflex arcs below the level of the lesion are isolated from higher centres. It usually increases in severity during the first few weeks after injury, after the period of spinal shock. In incomplete lesions it is often more pronounced and can be severe enough to prevent patients with good power in the legs from walking. Patients with severe spasticity and imbalance of opposing muscle groups have a tendency to develop contractures. It is important to realise that once a contracture occurs spasticity is increased and a vicious circle is established with further deformity resulting. Although excessive spasticity may hamper patients' activities or even throw them out of their wheelchairs or make walking impossible, spasticity may have advantages. It maintains muscle bulk and possibly bone density, and improves venous return.

Treatment of severe spasticity is indicated if it interferes with activities of daily living, and is initially directed at removing any obvious precipitating cause. An irritative lesion in the paralysed part, such as a pressure sore, urinary tract infection or calculus, anal fissure, infected ingrowing toenail, or fracture, tends to increase spasticity.

Passive stretching of spastic muscles and regular standing are helpful in relieving spasticity and preventing contractures. The drugs most commonly used to decrease spasticity are baclofen and tizanidine, which act at spinal level, and dantrolene sodium, which acts directly on skeletal muscle. Although diazepam relieves spasticity, its sedative action and habit-forming tendency limit its usefulness. With these drugs, the liver function tests need to be closely monitored.

If spasticity is localised it can be relieved by interrupting the nerve supply to the muscles affected by neurectomy after a diagnostic block with a long-acting local anaesthetic (bupivacaine). For example, in patients with severe hip adductor spasticity obturator neurectomy is effective. Alternatively, motor point injections, initially with bupivacaine, followed by either 6% aqueous phenol or 45% ethyl alcohol for

---

Box 6.7 Factors that aggravate spasticity

- Urinary tract infection or calculus
- Infected ingrowing toenail
- Pressure sores
- Anal fissure
- Fracture
- Contractures

Box 6.8 Management of spasticity

- Treat factors that aggravate spasticity
- Improve comfort/posture
- Manage pain
- Passively stretch spastic muscles
- Regular standing
- Oral therapy—baclofen
  —tizanidine
  —dantrolene
  —diazepam
- Botulinum toxin
- Motor point injections
- Implanted drug delivery system for administration of intrathecal baclofen

If the above fail, are contraindicated, or are unavailable:
- tendon release and/or neurectomy, and other orthopaedic procedures
- intrathecal block (rarely used)—6% aqueous phenol
  —absolute alcohol

a more lasting effect, are useful in selected patients. Botulinum toxin also has a limited use in patients with localised spasticity.

If oral agents are failing to control generalised spasticity intrathecal baclofen will often provide relief. If a small test dose of 50 micrograms baclofen given by lumbar puncture relieves the spasticity, a reservoir and pump can be implanted to provide regular and long-term delivery of the drug. It is now rare to have to resort to destructive procedures involving surgical or chemical neurectomy, or intrathecal blocks with 6% aqueous phenol or absolute alcohol. The effect of phenol usually lasts a few months, that of alcohol is permanent. The main disadvantage in the use of either is that they convert an upper motor neurone to a lower motor neurone lesion and thus affect bladder, bowel, and sexual function.

Contractures

A contracture may be a result of immobilisation, spasticity, or muscle imbalance between opposing muscle groups. It may respond to conservative measures such as gradual stretching of affected muscles, often with the use of splints. If these measures fail to correct the deformity or are inappropriate, then surgical correction by tenotomy, tendon lengthening, or muscle division may be required. For example, a flexion contracture of the hip responds to an iliopsoas myotomy with division of the anterior capsule and soft tissues over the front of the joint.

Pressure sores

Pressure sores form as a result of ischaemia, caused by unrelieved pressure, particularly over bony prominences. They may affect not only the skin but also subcutaneous fat, muscle, and deeper structures. If near a joint, septic arthritis may supervene. The commonest sites are over the ischial tuberosity, greater trochanter, and sacrum. Pressure sores are a major cause of readmission to hospital, yet they are generally preventable by vigilance and recognition of simple principles.

Regular changes of position in bed every two to three hours and lifting in the wheelchair every 15 minutes are essential. A suitable mattress and wheelchair cushion are particularly important. The cushion should be selected for the individual patient after measuring the interface pressures between the ischial tuberosities and the cushion. Cushions need frequent checking and renewing if necessary. Shearing forces to the skin from underlying structures are avoided by correct lifting; the skin should never be dragged along supporting surfaces. Patients must not lie for long periods with the skin unprotected on x ray diagnostic units or on operating tables (in this situation Roho mattress sections placed under the patient are of benefit). A pressure clinic is extremely useful in checking the sitting posture, assessing the wheelchair and cushion, and generally instilling pressure consciousness into patients. If a red mark on the skin is noticed which does not fade within 20 minutes the patient should avoid all pressure on that area until the redness and any underlying induration disappears.

If an established sore is present, any slough is excised and the wound is dressed with a desloughing agent if necessary. Once the wound is clean and has healthy granulation tissue, occlusive dressings may be used. Complete relief of pressure on the affected area is essential until healing has occurred. Indications for surgery are: (1) a large sore which would take too long to heal using conservative methods; (2) a sore with infected bone in its base; (3) a discharging sinus with an underlying bursa. If possible, surgical treatment is by excision

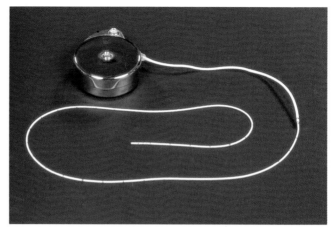

Figure 6.11 The Medtronic SynchroMed® EL infusion system consists of a programmable pump and catheter. The central fill port is used for the administration of intrathecal baclofen, and the side catheter access port is used for direct intrathecal access of other drugs or contrast, by-passing the pump.

Box 6.9 Treatment of contractures

- Gradual stretching ± splints
- Tenotomy
- Tendon lengthening
- Muscle and soft tissue division

Box 6.10 Prevention of pressure sores

- Regular relief of pressure
- Regular checking of skin, using mirror
- Avoid all pressure if red mark develops
- Suitable cushion and mattress, checked regularly
- Avoid tight clothes and hard seams

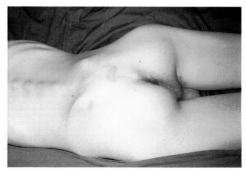

Figure 6.12 Pressure marks over sacrum and posterior iliac crests. Relief of pressure over these areas must be continued until marks have faded. In this patient this was achieved after only three days of bed rest with appropriate positioning.

of the sore and any underlying bony prominence, with direct closure in layers, leaving a small linear scar. Most pressure sores can be managed in this way. Recurrence is uncommon and if it occurs can be more easily treated after this type of surgery than if large areas of tissues have been disturbed by previous use of a flap.

Further reading

- An HS. *Principles and techniques of spine surgery*. Baltimore: Williams and Wilkins, 1998
- Ayers DC, McCollister Evarts C, Parkinson JR. The prevention of heterotopic ossification in high-risk patients by low-dose radiation therapy after total hip arthroplasty. *J Bone Joint Surg* 1986;**68A**:1423–30
- Errico TJ. Techniques and management of cervical spine fractures. In: Lorenz MA, ed. *Spine: state of the art reviews. Spinal fracture-dislocations*, vol 7. Philadelphia: Hanley and Belfus, 1993
- Karlsson AK. Autonomic dysreflexia. *Spinal Cord* 1999;**37**:383–91
- Schmidt SA, Kjaersgaard-Andersen, Pedersen NW, Kristensen SS, Pedersen P, Nielsen JB. The use of indomethacin to prevent the formation of heterotopic bone after total hip replacement. *J Bone Joint Surg* 1988;**70A**:834–8
- Tator CH, Duncan EG, Edmonds VE, Lapczak LI, Andrews DF. Neurological recovery, mortality and length of stay after acute spinal cord injury associated with changes in management. *Paraplegia* 1995;**33**:254–62

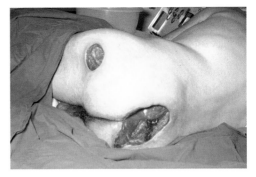

Figure 6.13 Extensive sacral and trochanteric pressure sores.

Box 6.11 Treatment of pressure sores

Conservative—complete relief of pressure
        —if slough, treat with desloughing agent or excise
        —treat general condition, e.g. correct anaemia
Surgical   —direct closure if possible, with removal of underlying
          bony prominence

7 Urological management

Peter Guy, David Grundy

After spinal cord injury (SCI), dysfunctional voiding patterns soon emerge. These are usually characterised by hyperreflexic bladder contractions in suprasacral cord lesions and acontractile bladders in conus medullaris and cauda equina lesions. Quite apart from socially incapacitating incontinence, the resulting urodynamic abnormalities can lead to recurrent urinary tract infection (UTI), vesico-ureteric reflux, and upper tract dilatation and hydronephrosis. This results in long-term damage to the urinary tract, with eventual renal failure. Constant urological vigilance is therefore an essential part of management.

Early management

Intermittent catheterisation

Ideally, intermittent catheterisation begins on arrival in the spinal injuries unit, using a size 12–14 lubricated Nelaton catheter. Commercially available coated self-lubricating catheters are now widely available. Catheterisation is undertaken 4–6 hourly; by restricting fluid intake to maintain a urine output of around 1500 ml per day, bladder volumes should not exceed 400–500 ml per catheterisation.

Most patients will, however, have had a standard Foley catheter inserted at the admitting emergency department, often to measure hourly urine output as part of the general management of the seriously injured patient.

In practice, many will retain an indwelling catheter until about 12 weeks after injury, when formal urodynamic appraisal can be undertaken. Definitive bladder management can then be planned and initiated.

Tapping and expression

After a period of "spinal shock", involuntary detrusor activity is observed in most patients with suprasacral cord lesions. By about 12 weeks after injury, those patients who it is felt may manage without long-term catheters will have begun bladder training. In those with minimal detrusor-distal sphincter dyssynergia (DSD see below), suprapubic tapping and, if necessary, compression may be sufficient to empty the bladder. Tapping and compression continue until urinary flow ceases. The process is repeated every 2 hours.

When male patients begin to void, they wear condom sheaths attached to urinary drainage bags. Their fluid intake is no longer restricted, and the frequency of intermittent catheterisation is gradually reduced. Initially, the post "voiding" residual volume is checked daily, either by "in-out" catheters, or using a portable bladder scanner. When this is <100 ml on three consecutive occasions, bladder training is complete, and intermittent catheterisation is discontinued. The residual volume requires re-checking during the first year.

Indwelling catheterisation

In those patients unsuited to tapping and expression or intermittent self-catheterisation (ISC), consideration may be given to long-term indwelling catheterisation as a permanent method of bladder drainage.

Box 7.1 Aims of management

- Preservation of renal function
- Continence

Box 7.2 Intermittent urethral catheterisation

- Clean technique
- 6-hourly programme
- Fluid restriction
- Treat significant UTI

Box 7.3 Complications of urethral catheters

- Infection
    Epididymo-orchitis
    Paraurethral gland abscess
    Urethral diverticulum/fistula
- Calculous/biofilm encrustation
- Recurrent blockage +/− dysreflexic attacks
- Urethral erosion (females)
- Traumatic hypospadias (males)

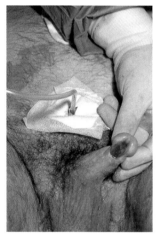

Figure 7.1 Catheter complications: traumatic hypospadias in a paraplegic, associated with a urethral catheter, and requiring change to suprapubic drainage.

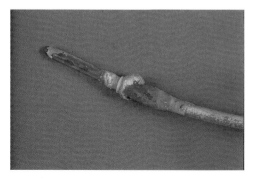

Figure 7.2 Catheter complications: encrustation.

Both short- and long-term indwelling catheters are convenient, but have risks and complications. Wheelchair-bound female patients with urethral catheters are especially prone to urethral erosion and such patients (especially if they have hyperreflexic bladders) are unsuitable for long-term urethral catheters, once they have mobilised. Women with strong bladder contractions may expel both balloon and catheter, causing a severe dilatation of the urethra. Early suprapubic catheterisation should be considered in this group.

In men, pressure necrosis at the external urethral meatus causes an increasing traumatic hypospadias and cleft penile urethra.

Urethral catheters should be as small as is compatible with good drainage, and should preferably be made of pure silicone. These catheters may be left in situ for 6–8 weeks.

Wherever possible, regular "cycling" of the bladder should take place, using a catheter valve to intermittently release urine. This helps to maintain bladder volume and compliance, though where detrusor activity is present, anticholinergic therapy is indicated. This is particularly important where the patient may be deemed eventually suitable for ISC.

Patients with indwelling catheters are prone to develop calculous blockage, and bladder washouts with water, saline or Suby-G solution are recommended on a weekly basis, especially if the urine is cloudy with sediment. A fluid intake of 2.5–3 L per day may help reduce the risk of calculous blockage and infection. Regular blockage should be investigated with cystoscopy and removal of any stone fragments.

Urine is cultured weekly, and at other times if indicated. *Proteus* sp. and *Klebsiella* are urea splitting organisms, and particularly important bacteria to eradicate. These infections and the resulting alkalisation are associated with a high incidence of "struvite" stone (calcium apatite and magnesium ammonium phosphate) formation in both the bladder and the upper tracts. Stag-horn calculi require early removal by percutaneous or open pyelolithotomy, before the infected stone results in the development of xanthogranulomatous pyelonephritis and an inevitable nephrectomy. Percutaneous dissolution of struvite stone (e.g. with hemiacidrin) is sometimes successful.

Catheterised patients invariably develop colonised urine, usually with a mixed flora. Antibiotic therapy is not indicated here, unless the patient develops systemic signs of infection (including skin "marking").

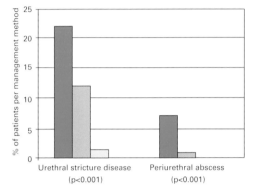

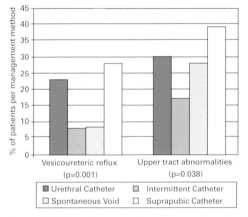

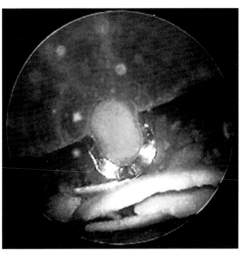

Figure 7.3 Complications of long-term catheterisation. Weld KJ, Dmochowski RR. Effect of bladder management on urological complications in spinal cord injured patients. *J Urol* 2000;**163**:768–72. Reproduced with permission.

Suprapubic catheterisation (SPC)

Patients with large acontractile bladders (capacity >500 ml) can be safely catheterised on the ward under local anaesthetic and cystodistension, using one of the commercially available introducing trocars and a 12 or 16 Ch Foley catheter. The poor "balloon memory" of pure silicone catheters may cause difficulty with subsequent removal, and coated latex may be the material of choice for suprapubic catheters. Care should be taken in selecting an appropriate suprapubic puncture site to avoid deep skin creases. In obese patients, and in those with small and hyperreflexic bladders, careful cystoscopic placement of the stab cystostomy trocar, or formal open cystostomy under general or spinal anaesthesia in the operating room is recommended. In this way, autonomic dysreflexia is avoided, and the risk of inadvertent small bowel injury is minimised.

SPC is increasingly used as a method of bladder drainage in the first few weeks after SCI, and is the personal preference of many patients in the long term. Fluid restriction is unnecessary—an intake of 3 litres per day may help reduce the risk of blockage.

Figure 7.4 Catheter complications: egg shell calculus.

Although SPC avoids risks to the urethra and allows greater sexual freedom, it shares many of the other unwanted side effects of permanent urethral catheterisation. Blockage by sediment, and in hyperreflexic patients, by lumenal compression and mucosal plugging results in "bypassing", and in high cord lesions, the associated bladder spasm frequently results in episodes of autonomic dysreflexia.

Intermittent self-catheterisation (ISC)

When intermittent catheterisation has been performed by the nursing staff as part of initial bladder management, ISC can start as soon as the patient sits up. Patients catheterise themselves with the aim of remaining continent between catheterisations, therefore avoiding the need to wear urinary drainage apparatus.

Patients with acontractile bladders are the most suitable candidates for ISC, though hyperreflexic detrusor activity is not a contraindication provided it is well controlled with anticholinergic therapy.

A "clean" but not sterile technique is employed, using 12–14 Ch Nelaton catheters. Although commercially available coated single use catheters are popular in hospitals, Nelaton catheters with applied lubricating gel are significantly cheaper in the community. There is a small risk of urethral trauma and subsequent stricture associated with re-usable catheters. However, patients appear no more vulnerable to infection by using such catheters, and in developing countries (provided they can be washed in clean water) re-usable catheters should be the first choice.

The long-term results of ISC compare favourably with other forms of bladder management, and the incidence of infection and stone formation is considerably less than in those patients with long-term indwelling catheters.

Investigations and urological review

Radiology

Ultrasound (US)

This is the most useful non-invasive technique to monitor bladder emptying and the integrity of the upper tracts. The combination of plain abdominal radiography with US has superseded routine intravenous urography for annual review, and most of the important changes to the upper tracts, especially dilatation, parenchymal scarring, and stone formation, can be diagnosed on US. When abnormalities are detected, other imaging modalities may be required.

Video-urodynamics

Although the degree of detrusor activity may be predicted by the level of the SCI, formal baseline studies should be performed at 3–4 months to enable definitive bladder management to be planned. The investigation is in two parts. The cystometrogram relates the filling pressure to bladder volumes, and identifies and quantifies unstable contractions and abnormalities of compliance. The simultaneous contrast radiological study allows screening of the bladder and urethra. This is an important part of the investigation and is video-recorded or the images digitised. In many patients with a suprasacral cord lesion, detrusor contractions are associated with a simultaneous contraction of the distal sphincter mechanism—the void is obstructed due to the "dyssynergic"

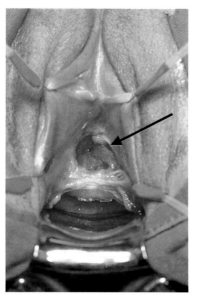

Figure 7.5 Catheter complications: female urethral erosion.

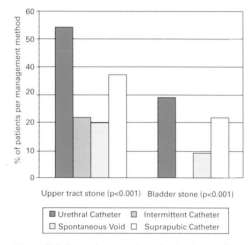

Figure 7.6 Intermittent catheterisation is associated with fewer urinary stones. Weld KJ. Reproduced with permission.

Box 7.4 Optimum requirements for intermittent self-catheterisation

- Minimal detrusor activity
- Large capacity bladder
- Adequate outlet resistance
- Manual dexterity
- Pain-free catheterisation
- Patient motivation

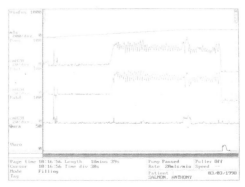

Figure 7.7 Cystometrogram showing sustained detrusor contractions.

distal sphincter. Dyssynergic high pressure voiding frequently causes autonomic dysreflexia, a potentially serious and occasionally fatal autonomic disturbance resulting in severe hypertension. It is discussed in detail in chapter 6. Although the distal sphincter eventually relaxes, the unstable "voiding" detrusor contraction usually fades away before the bladder has emptied properly, leaving a significant residual. This encourages infection and stone formation, and ongoing unstable contractions often lead to vesico-ureteric reflux, hydronephrosis, and pyelonephritis. The contrast part of the study helps characterise many aspects of these extremely important complications, and enables appropriate (often surgical) action to be taken before irreparable damage takes place.

Isotope renography/nuclear medicine

DMSA renography is a sensitive indicator of renal scarring and differential renal function, and is indicated when US studies suggest upper tract damage. DTPA and MAG 3 renography are useful investigations to characterise upper tract obstruction, and also to monitor the progress of the kidney after treatment for vesico-ureteric reflux. Serial estimation of the glomerular filtration rate (GFR) using Cr-EDTA or Tc-DTPA is a sensitive method of determining any decline in renal function, and a reduction in GFR (or creatinine clearance) is observed before changes can be measured in serum creatinine.

Biochemistry

Routine baseline serum creatinine, urea and electrolyte estimations are performed, and should be repeated annually until the clinician in charge is certain that the urinary tract is completely stable on definitive management, and with no significant radiological or urodynamic prognostic risk factors.

Later management

In many patients the early management of the urinary tract merges with the long-term plan. With the increasing use of suprapubic catheters at an initial stage, many tetraplegic patients are discharged into the community content not to alter this method of bladder management. However, both suprapubic and urethral catheters should be discouraged where safer methods are available, especially in paraplegics. Above all, the merits of ISC should be stressed to the patient. In those men whose penis will retain a condom, sheath drainage is an extremely safe method of bladder management. Where necessary, endoscopic distal sphincterotomy is undertaken to abolish dyssynergia.

Personal choice is now emerging as a major factor in planning, and the individual's lifestyle preferences must be taken account of, though not at the expense of risk to the upper tracts. Some aspire to continence and freedom from indwelling catheters. Others are unwilling to self-catheterise, and will not relinquish their suprapubic catheters. Tetraplegics with poor hand function have fewer choices available to them, and avoidance of autonomic dysreflexia and freedom from infection may be the dominating influences in their personal choice.

After the first year, many paraplegic and a few incomplete tetraplegic patients wish to explore alternatives that allow freedom from permanent catheterisation, and restoration of continence. Patient awareness and lifestyle aspirations are increasing the demand for complex lower urinary tract reconstruction. Surgical options are tailored for each individual, and the urologist advising spinally damaged patients

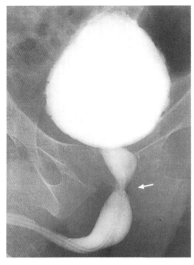

Figure 7.8 Detrusor-distal sphincter dyssynergia.

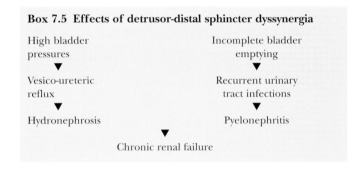

Box 7.5 Effects of detrusor-distal sphincter dyssynergia

High bladder pressures
▼
Vesico-ureteric reflux
▼
Hydronephrosis

Incomplete bladder emptying
▼
Recurrent urinary tract infections
▼
Pyelonephritis

▼
Chronic renal failure

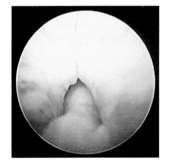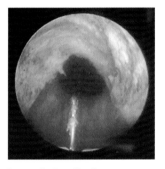

Figure 7.9 Endoscopic appearance, before and after distal sphincterotomy.

Box 7.6 Isotope renography in spinal cord injury

DMSA: Differential renal function
    Renal scarring
    Accurate and reproducible in long-term follow-up
Tc-DTPA and MAG3: Diagnosis and follow-up of uretero-pelvic junction or ureteral obstruction
    Indirect cystography for vesico-ureteric reflux
    Differential renal function
    Indirect measurement of GFR
Cr-EDTA GFR: Serial assay is a sensitive index of small changes in GFR

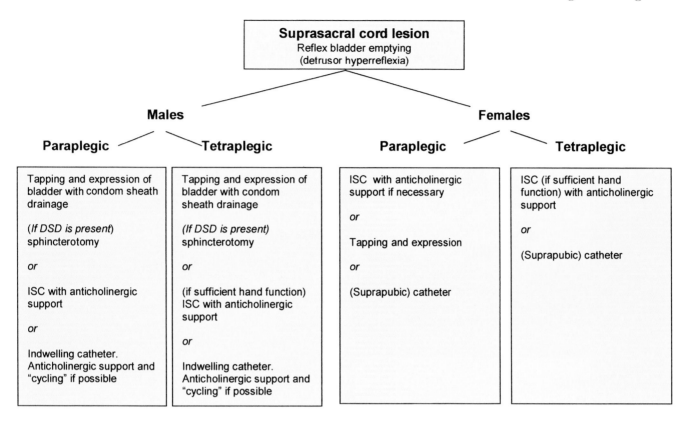

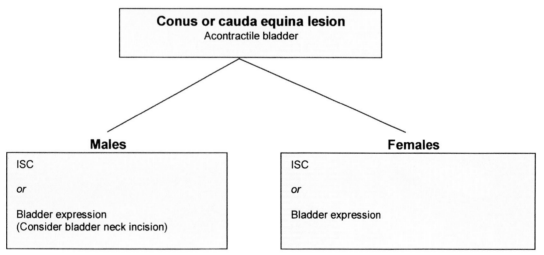

Figure 7.10 Later management changes: algorithms of basic bladder management.

must balance the potential to improve symptoms against unrealistic patient expectations and the possibility of surgical complications.

Simultaneous faecal incontinence and female pelvic floor disorders (especially following cauda eqina lesions) frequently require a multidisciplinary approach. In particular, the involvement of specialist nurse practitioners and stomatherapists at an early stage in planning treatment is emphasised.

Detrusor hyperreflexia

In the presence of DSD, sustained rises in detrusor pressure (P_{det}) may result in severe renal damage secondary to obstruction or high pressure vesico-ureteric reflux of (infected)

Box 7.7 Detrusor hyperreflexia in the presence of DSD

Risks:
- Autonomic dysreflexia in patients with spinal cord lesions above T6
- Renal damage due to
  —obstruction
  —high pressure vesico-ureteric reflux

urine. Continence and voiding are secondary considerations in these cases (nearly always males), where renal preservation is of the utmost priority. Recurrent suprapubic catheter blockage is common, even in the absence of calculous debris, and may result from catheter shaft compression by grossly unstable bladder contractions and mucosal plugging. Significant rises in detrusor pressure may occur even in the presence of an indwelling catheter on free drainage, and an association between these unstable contractions and upper tract scarring has recently been confirmed. Suprapubic catheters (SPC) should be cycled on at least two occasions each day, and simultaneous anticholinergic therapy should be used. Some men may opt for distal endoscopic sphincterotomy or stenting and condom drainage rather than SPC. Stents are less reliable in SCI patients than in those with outflow obstruction associated with prostatic enlargement. Others may be obese or suffer penile retraction, and condom sheath drainage may be impossible.

The maintenance of continence is of vital importance to personal morale, and for the preservation of intact perineal and buttock skin. We briefly examine some of the many surgical procedures available to restore continence and to facilitate self-catheterisation.

Augmentation cystoplasty

Where conventional medical treatment with anticholinergic therapy has failed, and if indwelling catheters are to be avoided, the bladder must be deafferentated or bisected and augmented with a patch of bowel to provide a bladder of sufficient compliance and volume to safely accommodate a socially useful volume of urine. In female patients, DSD is very unusual, and severe incontinence rather than upper tract protection is the main indication for augmentation. After augmentation, inability to void is the rule rather than the exception, and the patient must demonstrate the willingness and ability to self-catheterise before surgery can be contemplated.

Even after augmentation, anticholinergic therapy may be required to make the patient completely dry. Cystitis may be a recurrent problem after enterocystoplasty, and there remains a long-term theoretical risk of neoplastic transformation in the enteric patch, especially if this is colon. Nitrosamine production associated with UTI has been implicated in this process.

For those who cannot access their own urethra (wheelchair-bound females being an especially important group), the simultaneous provision of a self-catheterising abdominal stoma (Mitrofanoff) may be an integral part of the initial surgery (see below).

Neuromodulation and sacral anterior root stimulation (SARS)

In patients with complete suprasacral cord lesions, functional electrical stimulation of the anterior nerve roots of S2, S3 and S4 is very successful in completely emptying the paralysed bladder. Assisted defaecation, and in the male, implant-induced erections may be coincidental advantages of the implant. The device most commonly in use is the Finetech-Brindley stimulator; the anterior roots of S2, S3 and S4 are stimulated via a receiver block implanted under the skin, and a posterior rhizotomy is performed simultaneously. This cures reflex incontinence, improves bladder compliance and diminishes DSD, and thus ensures that neither the use of the implant nor overfilling of the bladder will trigger autonomic dysreflexia. Reflex erections and ejaculation will be lost with posterior

Box 7.8 Detrusor hyperreflexia: medical management

- Anticholinergic treatment
  Oxybutynin
  Tolterodine
  Propiverine HCl
  Flavoxate
  Propantheline
- Intravesical therapy (experimental)
  Capsaicin
  Resiniferatoxin

Box 7.9 Detrusor hyperreflexia: surgical management

- Augmentation cystoplasty
- Sacral anterior root stimulator (SARS)
- Posterior rhizotomy
- Urinary diversion

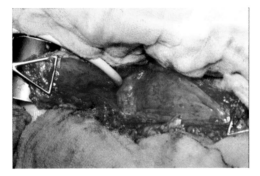

Figure 7.11 Illustration of the two halves of the bisected bladder ("clammed") prior to augmentation.

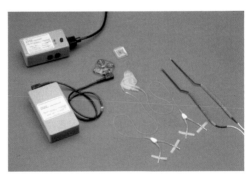

Figure 7.12 Components of the Finetech-Brindley SARS.

rhizotomy, and simultaneous neuromodulation is under investigation as an alternative to rhizotomy in men.

No comparative or controlled prospective studies between augmentation cystoplasty and SARS are yet available, but despite its cost, the stimulator is amongst the first in a line of options designed to keep this group of patients catheter free.

Stress incontinence

Both male and female patients with conus and cauda equina lesions are vulnerable to sphincter weakness incontinence (SWI), as well as older women with pre-existing pelvic floor disorders, prolapse, etc. regardless of the neurological level of injury. This often manifests itself later as the patient becomes more active during rehabilitation, urinary leakage occurring for example on transfer to and from the wheelchair.

Colposuspension, pubo-urethral slings and, recently, tension free vaginal tapes are effective in treating SWI, though sometimes obstructive in patients with acontractile bladders attempting to void by straining or compression. In paraplegic females, urethral closure and SPC is a reliable method of ensuring continence, though where appropriate, permanent suprapubic catheterisation may be avoided by performing a Mitrofanoff procedure. Bladder neck injections with bulking agents have a less reliable record in this difficult group.

Artificial urinary sphincters (AUS) have an excellent record of continence, but there is a higher attrition rate in paraplegics due to infection or cuff erosion, especially if ISC is undertaken regularly. Placement around the bulbar urethra should be avoided in patients confined to a wheelchair, and impotence frequently complicates cuff placement in the membranous position. For both male and female paraplegic patients the bladder neck is therefore the optimal site for AUS cuff placement.

The acontractile bladder and assisted voiding

Since the adoption and widespread use of intermittent self-catheterisation (ISC) in detrusor failure the complications of chronic retention and long-term catheterisation have been significantly reduced. Most patients with good hand function manage the technique, though paraplegic females have more difficulty accessing their urethra. This may be sufficient to cause them to abandon attempts in favour of long-term suprapubic catheterisation.

Since Mitrofanoff first described his technique in children, the procedure has been adapted to other circumstances, including stomal intermittent self-catheterisation in the paraplegic wheelchair-bound female patient. Even in tetraplegic patients with limited hand function stomal ISC is sometimes feasible with careful siting of the channel. In those patients who have undergone a Mitrofanoff procedure, stomal ISC is usually regarded as preferable to urethral catheterisation, and females whose native urethra remains *in situ* and who have a stoma almost never catheterise their own urethra. Complications of the procedure are irritatingly frequent though rarely life-threatening. Minor "plastic" procedures for stomal stenosis are required in up to 30% of cases and complete channel revisions for leakage or failure are necessary in 15%.

The procedure may be undertaken in conjunction with bladder augmentation and/or bladder neck closure for intractable incontinence.

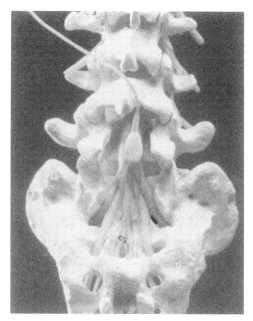

Figure 7.13 SARS: position of stimulating electrodes after laminectomy.

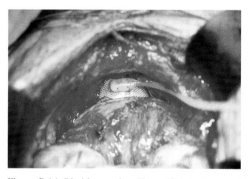

Figure 7.14 Bladder neck cuff—artificial urinary sphincter.

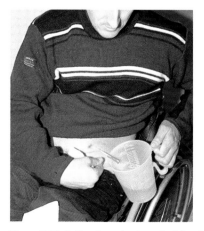

Figure 7.15 Self-catheterisation of a Mitrofanoff stoma.

Mixed faecal and urinary incontinence

Cauda equina lesions causing sphincter weakness frequently result in mixed faecal and urinary incontinence. This may have a devastating impact on rehabilitation, and the urologist should not consider involuntary urinary loss in isolation. Malone described the effectiveness of the antegrade colonic (continence) enema (ACE) in children with meningomyelocoele, and it may be helpful in managing sphincter weakness faecal incontinence secondary to cauda equina or conus injury. The procedure (like the Mitrofanoff) consists of the construction of a self-catheterising channel from appendix or tapered small bowel between abdominal wall and underlying caecum or colon. Every 48 hours or thereabouts, the bowel is intubated via the stoma, and a large volume enema (e.g. 2 L water) administered to wash the bowel clear of faeces. Continence is achieved until the large bowel refills. The ACE procedure is much less effective in treating the profound constipation frequently encountered in suprasacral SCI. The procedure can be performed simultaneous to a Mitrofanoff, colposuspension, urethral closure, or bladder neck cuff implantation, although the remaining components of the AUS should not be implanted due to the risk of infection.

Further reading

- Christensen P, Kvitzau B, Krogh K *et al*. Neurogenic colorectal dysfunction—use of the new antegrade and retrograde colonic wash-out methods. *Spinal Cord* 2000;**38**:255–61
- Galloway A. Prevention of urinary tract infection in patients with spinal cord injury—a microbiological review. *Spinal Cord* 1997;**35**:198–204
- Giannantoni A, Scivoletto G, Di Stasi SM *et al*. Clean intermittent catheterisation and the prevention of renal disease in spinal cord injury. *Spinal Cord* 1998;**36**:29–32
- Kelly SR, Shashidharan M, Borwell B *et al*. The role of intestinal stoma in patients with spinal cord injury. *Spinal Cord* 1999;**37**:211–14
- Sheriff MKM, Foley S, McFarlane J *et al*. Long term suprapubic catheterisation: clinical outcome and satisfaction survey. *Spinal Cord* 1998;**36**:171–6
- Sutton MA, Hinson JL, Nickell KG, Boone TB. Continent ileocecal augmentation cystoplasty. *Spinal Cord* 1998;**36**:246–51
- Weld KJ, Dmochowski RR. Effect of bladder management on urological complications in spinal cord injured patients. *J Urol* 2000;**163**:768–72

8   Nursing

Catriona Wood, Elizabeth Binks, David Grundy

The main nursing objectives in providing care for people who have sustained a spinal cord lesion are to: identify problems and prevent deterioration; prevent secondary complications; facilitate maximal functional recovery; support patients and significant others in learning to adjust to the patients' changed physical status; be aware of the effect of the injury on the patients' perception of self worth; give high priority to empowering patients, enabling them to take control of their life through formal and informal education.

Nurses need to recognise that patients will spend a long time in hospital, probably between four and nine months. Most patients are male (4:1 men to women) aged between 15 and 40 years, but an increasing number of older people are sustaining injuries. Patients will initially be very dependent on others, and those with high lesions or from the older age group may continue to be dependent and have a disappointing level of neurological recovery and functional outcome.

Factors which contribute to establishing close and supportive relationships between staff and patients often blur boundaries between professional and personal roles. This, with the psychological support required by patients, and the increased need for physical input, offers many challenges, yet many rewards to the nurse involved in care.

The psychological trauma of spinal cord injury is profound and prolonged. The impact on the injured person and his or her family is highly individual and varies from patient to patient throughout the course of their care. Fear and anxiety, worsened by sensory deprivation, may initially be considerable and continue in some degree for many months. During the acute phase, particularly when patients are confined to bed, they may experience a wide variety of mood swings including anger, depression, and euphoria. They may exhibit behaviour identifiable with a normal grieving process—guilt, denial or other coping mechanisms such as regression. They may suffer from a sense of frustration, be verbally demanding, or sometimes withdrawn.

Relatives often progress to adjustment much more quickly than the patients themselves, and this may complicate planning for the future. Intervention must take into consideration the coping mechanisms used by the patients and their families. Long-term decisions must not be taken before patients are willing and able to participate.

Certain landmarks in rehabilitation are especially stressful for the patient. Any occasion experienced for the first time after injury is likely to be psychologically demanding. Being mobilised from bed to wheelchair is one example, with its combination of blood pressure instability, physical exhaustion, and the shock of coming to terms with altered body sensation and image. For many, visits to home and friends are other physical and psychological hurdles that must be crossed. Most spinal injuries units have an "aid to daily living" (ADL) flat, where patients and their carer can stay prior to their first weekend at home, with staff close at hand if problems arise.

These events need careful preparation, with discussion taking place before and afterwards, initially with staff from the unit, and later with family and friends. Discharge from hospital is a considerable challenge, with patients and their families often having to cope with lack of stamina; loneliness; social isolation, and the changed relationship caused by injury. Continuing support will be needed for at least two to three years while the patient adjusts to his or her new lifestyle.

Box 8.1 Nursing aims

- Identify problems and prevent deterioration
- Prevent secondary complications
- Maximise functional recovery
- Support patients and relatives
- Empower patients
- Educate patients to take control of their lives.

Box 8.2 Psychological trauma

- Fear and anxiety
- Sensory deprivation
- Wide variety of moods
- Behaviour similar to the grieving process.

Box 8.3 Stressful rehabilitation landmarks

- Any occasion experienced for the first time
- Visits home to family and friends
- Discharge

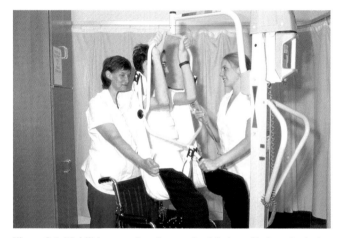

Figure 8.1 Mobilising a patient into a wheelchair—offering physical and psychological support.

Nursing management

In the emergency department

Many patients arrive in the emergency department from the scene of an accident on a spinal board, which enables the paramedics to immobilise the back or neck, and maintain spinal alignment. If a cervical spine injury is suspected, and no collar has been applied, the neck should be immobilised by using a semirigid collar supplemented with sandbags or bolsters taped to the forehead and collar, except in the case of the physically uncooperative or thrashing patient (see chapter 2). In an ideal situation, the collar must remain in place until completion of the initial assessment, resuscitation, and diagnostic x rays. The decision to remove the collar must be made by a competent member of the medical team.

The non-conforming nature of the spinal board means that potential pressure points are exposed to high interface pressures. This necessitates removal of the spinal board as soon as is appropriate by a coordinated trained team. With the neck held, and with the use of a log roll, the patient should be transferred using a sliding board on to a well-padded trauma trolley with a firm base, in case resuscitation is needed. If resuscitation or the insertion of an airway is necessary, the chin lift or jaw thrust manoeuvre and not a head tilt is used for unconscious patients and those with suspected cervical spine lesions.

All clothing should be removed to facilitate full examination and inspection for skin damage. Care should be taken not to raise both of the arms above head level, to reduce the risk of cord lesion extension. Upper thoracic and cervical cord lesion patients may become poikilothermic (taking on the surrounding environmental temperature), with a tendency towards hypothermia. During the assessment phase, and their time in the emergency department, care must be taken to maintain the patient's temperature within acceptable levels.

Once a spinal cord injury has been diagnosed, care of pressure areas is extremely important. If delay in admission to the ward, where the patient will be nursed on a pressure-relieving mattress, is expected, the patient must be log rolled into the lateral position for one minute every hour. A firm mattress is more supportive to the spine, and far more comfortable.

In the acute and rehabilitation care setting

A patient-centred approach is essential to meet the various problems with which a patient may present. In the initial acute phase, nursing care will be implemented to meet the patient's own inability to maintain his or her own activities of daily living. As the patient progresses through the rehabilitation phase, the nurse's role becomes more supportive and educative, with the patient taking responsibility through self-care or by directing carers.

Choice of bed

The standard King's Fund bed, or profiling bed, with a stable mattress consisting of layers of varying density foam, is suitable for most patients, with the addition of a Balkan beam and spreader bar. It is probably the best bed for tetraplegics requiring skull traction, facilitating good positioning of the shoulders and arms. An electrically powered turning and tilting bed is particularly suitable for heavy patients, and those with multiple injuries. It facilitates postural drainage in chest injuries. It permits easier nursing as far as numbers are concerned, but still requires a full team of five or four nurses for inspection of pressure points, especially the natal cleft, for hygiene requirements, and bowel management.

Box 8.4 Emergency management

- Immobilisation of the neck
- Co-ordinated team
- Remove from spinal board
- Remove clothing
- Examine skin for marking and damage
- Pressure relief

Box 8.5 Hypothermia

High lesion patients are poikilothermic, therefore risk of hypothermia, with:
- Confusion
- Bradycardia ⇨ cardiac arrhythmias
- Hypoventilation
- Hypotension

Patient centred interdisciplinary approach

Essential throughout all stages of rehabilitation

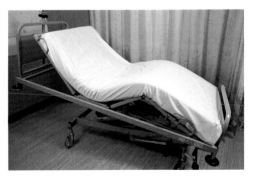

Figure 8.2 Profiling bed.

Positioning

Regular position changing is every two to three hours initially to relieve pressure. Skin inspection for red marks, spinal alignment and positioning of limbs is essential for a patient with spinal cord injury. The aims are simple: to support the injured spine in a good healing position; to maintain limbs and joints in a functional position, thus avoiding deformity and contractures, and to reduce the incidence of spasticity. There are several ways of achieving these aims, so the methods chosen should follow discussion with the interdisciplinary team, and suit the patient, level of injury, and the availability, knowledge and skill of the nursing staff.

Spinal alignment

Before undertaking a turn or preparing to move/transfer a patient, spinal alignment should be maintained by checking (when the patient is supine) that the nose, sternum and symphysis pubis are in alignment and that the shoulders and hips are level. A shoulder hold provides countertraction by applying pressure onto the shoulders to prevent an upward movement.

Handling and turning

Patient handling techniques need to be considered in relation to the Manual Handling Operations Regulations 1992. Patients with spinal cord injury are unable to help, and care must be taken to maintain alignment and stability of the neck and back at all times throughout the handling technique. This may pose problems for the staff when considering the method of transfer and movement of a patient, hence the need for rigorous assessment with the application of ergonomic principles.

Manual hoisting aids with stretcher attachments, and side to side, and up and down transfer products are available in the United Kingdom. Outside the European Community, and especially in developing countries, handling equipment may not be available, and there may be no alternatives following risk assessment but to handle the patient manually.

When transferring or moving a patient with an acute cervical injury, to maintain neck alignment and stability, the "lead" nurse holds the neck and head with both hands under the neck, and both wrists supporting the patient's head behind the ears (Figure 8.3). The nurse at the patient's head takes control and coordinates the turn after checking her team is ready.

Countertraction, starting at the top of the patient, may also be used to prevent movement of the spine when inserting hands or equipment under the patient, or starting at the foot end first when hands are being withdrawn (Figure 8.4).

A log roll is needed for carrying out nursing care, such as bowel management, skin hygiene, and for lateral positioning of both paraplegic and tetraplegic patients. Figure 8.5 shows how the paraplegic patient should be held when preparing to turn. Note the injury site is well supported. When the log roll is complete, the patient remains supported by pillows (Figure 8.6). Note the alignment of the shoulders, hip, iliac crest, and upper leg in Figure 8.6. A tetraplegic patient will require a head hold to complete this move. The nurse performing the head hold coordinates the manoeuvre. End positioning of the head will be determined by the mechanism of injury and the head and neck will be maintained in a neutral, extended, or flexed position, using a "water bag", neck roll, sand bag, or pillows.

Box 8.6 Acute phase

- Support injured spine in alignment
- Maintain limbs and joints in functional position
- Passive movements

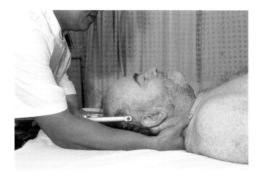

Figure 8.3 Head hold with head and neck supported by nurse's forearm and hands.

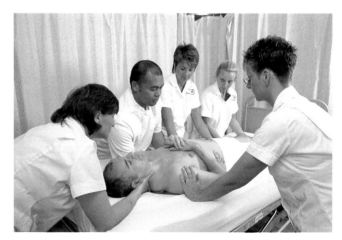

Figure 8.4 Countertraction to prevent movement of the spine.

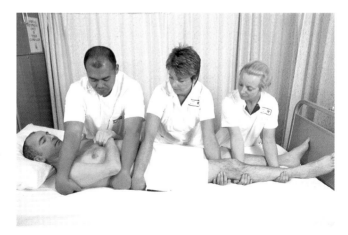

Figure 8.5 Preparing to log roll a paraplegic patient. For tetraplegic patient, a head hold is also needed.

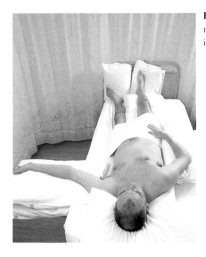

Figure 8.6 Completed log roll in a high thoracic injury in the lateral position.

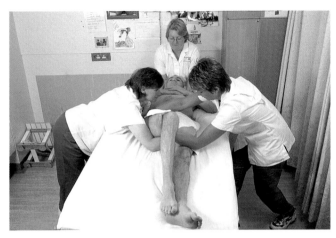

Figure 8.7 Preparing to pelvic twist.

The pelvic twist

The pelvic twist is a simple turn needing only three nurses to perform and suitable for many tetraplegic patients. It must not be used for patients with thoracolumbar lesions. The nurse at the patient's head holds the shoulders securely to the bed; the second nurse (standing on the side to which the patient is being turned), applies countertraction and gets ready to support the back and legs on completion of the twist, before inserting the pillows. The third nurse proceeds with the twist by placing her or his upper arm under the patient's back (using countertraction), and her or his lower arm under the patient's nearest thigh, and over the furthest thigh to support and move the hip. The movement is a gentle lift and turn of the near hip joint, enough to free the sacrum of any pressure (Figure 8.7). On completion of the turn, a pillow is folded in half into the lumbar region to support the back and pelvis, and two pillows are placed under the upper leg (Figures 8.8 and 8.9).

In all turns involving tetraplegic patients, the nurse holding the head is in charge of the timing and coordination of the team. The frequency of turns in the acute stage of management is determined by the patient's tolerance, but length between turns should not be greater than three hours.

Once the patient has progressed into the rehabilitation phase of care, the interval between turns can be increased, as long as there is no skin marking. The number of pillows used to support the body and limbs may be decreased.

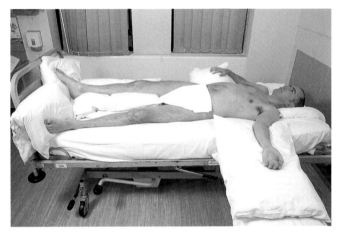

Figure 8.8 Pelvic twist completed, side/front view.

Legs

When patients are supine, avoid hyperextension of the knees. Keep the feet in line with the hips and hold the feet at 90° using a foot board and pillows. Avoid pressure on the heels.

When patients are on their side, the lower leg should be extended, with the upper leg slightly flexed and resting on pillows, and not over the lower leg.

Arms

When tetraplegic patients are supine, between turns, their joints need to be placed gently through a full range of positions to prevent stiffness and contractures. Hands and arms must always be supported through the movement. If remaining in

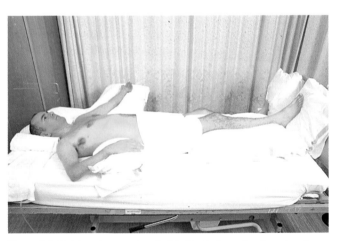

Figure 8.9 Pelvic twist completed: side/back view of patient showing folded pillow into small of back to maintain position—sacrum free of pressure.

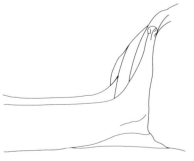

Figure 8.10 Heel is free of pressure with the foot held at 90°.

the supine position, arms and hands need to be supported down by the patient's side.

When positioning the patient in a left or right pelvic twist (see Figure 8.12), the arm facing the same direction as the twist can either be extended straight out (a), or the forearm placed pointing towards the head or downwards towards the feet (b). The forearm on the side away from the twist should point to the head or feet, but should not be in a similar position to the other arm (b).

In log rolls the lower arm is extended (a), with the upper arm placed at the patient's side, or flexed across the chest (b).

The shoulders and arms should always be protected from pressure—by gentle handling and good support with pillows.

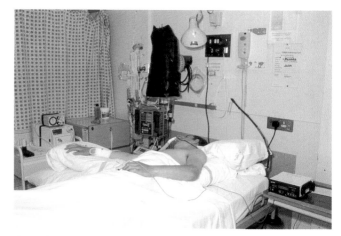

Figure 8.11 Monitoring the patient's internal environment in the acute phase.

Nursing intervention

Internal environment

Patients with high thoracic and cervical lesions are susceptible to respiratory complications, and a health education programme should be implemented with the long-term goal of reducing the risk of chest infections.

Monitoring in the acute phase should include skin colour, level of orientation, respiratory rate and depth, chest wall and diaphragmatic movement, oxygen saturation, chest auscultation, and vital capacity. Some patients will require additional oxygen therapy and possibly non-invasive pressure support. A physiotherapy programme will need to be continued throughout the 24-hour period with assisted coughing and bronchial and oral hygiene.

Cardiovascular monitoring will include not only the patient's blood pressure and pulse (high lesion patients may be hypotensive and bradycardic), but also observing for evidence

Box 8.7 Maintaining internal environment

- Respiration/support
- Assisted coughing
- Bronchial and oral hygiene
- Cardiovascular monitoring
- Antiembolism stockings
- Temperature control

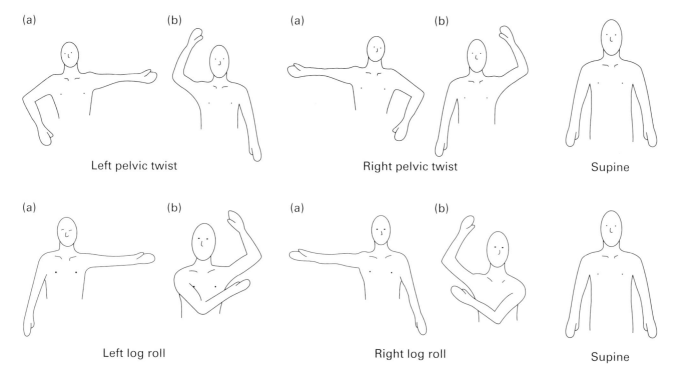

Left pelvic twist   Right pelvic twist   Supine

Left log roll   Right log roll   Supine

Figure 8.12 The arm positions (a) or (b) are changed as the patient is rotated through a turning regime of, for example:
Pelvic twist: left pelvic twist → right pelvic twist → supine.
or
Log roll: log roll to the left → log roll to the right → supine.
The turning regime will depend on the skin condition and comfort of the patient.

of deep vein thrombosis. As well as measuring the circumference of the calves and thighs, the patient's temperature must be monitored, as a low grade pyrexia is sometimes the only indication that thromboembolic complications are developing. Appropriately measured and fitted thigh-length antiembolism stockings should be applied.

The patient's body temperature should be maintained—high lesion patients are poikilothermic, and therefore hypothermia is a risk, particularly in cold weather.

Profound loss of sensation below the level of the lesion, a restricted visual field due to enforced bed rest, unfamiliar surroundings and many interruptions imposed on newly injured patients in the early stages may cause sensory deprivation leading to confusion and disorientation.

The imbalance can be redressed by increasing sensory input to the patient, but at the same time being careful not to overload the patient. Many tools can be used, one of which is that of touch, in a caring comforting manner, above the level of the lesion. Mirrors can be placed strategically to extend the field of vision and reality training employed by using clocks, calendars, newspapers, by using friends and relatives, and most importantly by allowing the patient to have a decision-making role.

Pain management

Pain management in the spinal cord injured patient is complex because of the various factors that can contribute towards the pain, both physical and emotional. Despite their paralysis, patients can still experience pain at the injury site. The use of a continuous infusion of opioids, normally subcutaneous, backed by the use of non-steroidal anti-inflammatory drugs usually provides satisfactory relief. Careful monitoring, including pulse oximetry, is necessary whilst the infusion is in use. Some patients develop shoulder pain, which needs to be managed with both physiotherapy and analgesia.

Skin hygiene and care

Skin cleanliness is fundamental, and good long-term arrangements for bathing or showering must be made. Minor skin infections should be treated and toe nails cut short and straight across, as ingrowing toe nails are particularly common. From an early stage, patients must be taught about the hazards of sensory loss and the need to inspect their skin and extremities regularly. They must be conscious of the effects of pressure and appreciate that the risk of pressure sores increases during times of emotional distress, tiredness, depression, and intercurrent illness.

Education is also important to enable the patient to select suitable clothing, with sore prevention and poikilothermia in mind.

Nutrition

Life-threatening conditions in the initial phase often overshadow the nutritional needs of the patient. The risk factors associated with trauma, the initial period of paralytic ileus, a reduced oral intake, anorexia and the inability to use the hands in high lesions, can all lead to malnutrition, skin complications, and severe weight loss. The nursing goal in the acute phase is to maintain nutritional support by: performing a nutritional risk assessment with the dietitian; implementing parenteral or enteral feeding when necessary; and encouraging and helping to feed the patient with their diet and nutritional supplements.

Box 8.8 Sensory deprivation

- Familiarisation of environment
- Interpretation of incoming stimuli
- Higher levels of cognitive functioning
- Reality orientation
- Decision-making role

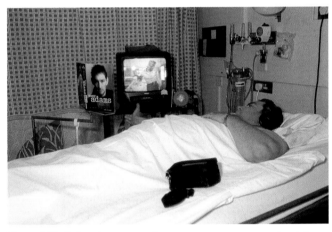

Figure 8.13 Enhancing sensory input to promote a more stimulating environment in the acute phase of spinal cord injury.

Box 8.9 Pain management

- Continuous infusion
- Non-steroidal anti-inflammatory drugs

Box 8.10 Skin care

- Avoid damage
- Educate regarding risks
- Examine and relieve pressure regularly
- Select suitable clothing
- Keep clean
- Treat minor abrasions/injuries

Box 8.11 Nutrition

- Nil by mouth initially
- Nutritional risk assessment
- Parenteral/enteral feeding
- Education:
    diet
    feeding aids

In the rehabilitation phase, the nurse needs to be familiar with feeding aids provided by the occupational therapist and to implement an individual education programme.

Bladder management

During the acute phase of spinal cord injury, bladder management involves strict fluid monitoring and insertion of an indwelling urethral or suprapubic catheter with, initially, hourly urine measurements.

The sudden hypotension in high lesions, and the large amounts of antidiuretic hormone secreted by the pituitary as a response to the stress of a major injury, leads to oliguria followed in some cases by a marked post-traumatic diuresis. It is important to prevent overdistention of the bladder during this stage, which could otherwise lead to overstretching of nerve endings and muscle fibres, inhibiting their potential to recover, which in turn could reduce the long-term management options for the patient.

The prevention of urinary tract infection through the implementation of good hygiene, adequate fluid intake and strict asepsis is vital.

The long-term aim is the prevention of complications such as urinary tract infections and calculi, as they may hinder a successful rehabilitation programme. Support and education by skilled staff enables the patient to make an informed choice as to the method of bladder management best suited to him/her, which in turn should improve the quality of life.

Catheterisation, either by the patient or carer, requires careful preparation and teaching, to provide the physical and psychological support necessary. Coming to terms with loss of this bodily function is often one of the hardest outcomes of SCI that the patient has to accept. Female patients provide an even greater challenge in the achievement of continence, because of "hormonal" leaking during the premenstrual and menstrual period, or a previous history of stress incontinence.

Long-term suprapubic catheterisation is now a popular method of management. It is sexually and aesthetically more acceptable, as well as reducing the risk of urethral damage associated with long-term urethral catheterisation. Patients and carers are taught to change their suprapubic catheters.

However, the use of long term indwelling catheters, either urethral or suprapubic, should not be generally recommended, because of the high incidence of side effects, including calculus formation and urinary tract infection. The presence of an indwelling catheter does not prevent upper urinary tract complications.

The temporary use of a suprapubic catheter with a catheter valve is an alternative to intermittent self-catheterisation as a method of training the bladder to empty reflexly.

If possible and practicable, intermittent self-catheterisation is considered one of the best methods of management. Careful control of fluids and a daily routine will be needed to maintain a dry state between catheters.

Emptying the bladder by tapping and expression, using condom sheath drainage, is also an excellent method in appropriate patients.

Part of the education is assisting the patient to adapt their chosen method into their individual lifestyle, as well as teaching the patient what to do if complications such as autonomic dysreflexia arise.

Bowel care

During the period of spinal shock, the bowel is flaccid, so it must not be allowed to overdistend, causing constipation with overflow incontinence. An initial rectal check is made to

---

Box 8.12 Bladder management – acute phase

- Strict fluid monitoring
- Avoidance of overdistension of bladder
- Strict asepsis and good hygiene

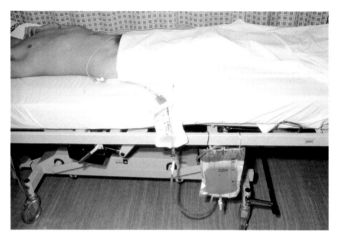

Figure 8.14 Bladder management—the use of a catheter valve within a suprapubic closed drainage system.

Box 8.13 Bladder management – long term aims

- Preservation of renal function
- Continence
- Prevention of infection, calculi and urethral trauma
- Appropriate fluid intake
- Informed choice of suitable bladder management programme
- Individual education package

Box 8.14 Bowel management

Upper motor neurone lesion:
- Reflex emptying—after suppositories or digital stimulation
- May not need aperients if diet appropriate

Lower motor neurone lesion:
- Flaccid
- Manual evacuation and aperients usually required but may be able to empty, using abdominal muscles
- Suppositories ineffective

Education
- Programme established to meet patient's lifestyle

ascertain whether faeces are present; if they are, they should be manually evacuated. Manual evacuation thereafter will continue daily or on alternate days. Very little bowel activity will be expected for the first two or three days. Evacuation should be performed using plenty of lubricant, and with only one gloved finger inserted into the anus. Trauma, including anal stretching and a split natal cleft, is possible if insufficient care is taken. Suppositories to lubricate or stimulate, possibly with the use of aperients, may be required to achieve an evacuation after the initial period of spinal shock. The patient is taught to have an adequate fibre diet, and a high fluid intake to help prevent constipation. The use of aperients is kept to a minimum, especially in a patient with reflex bowel activity. The use of natural laxatives is encouraged in the diet.

Slowly a routine is established that will fit into the patient's future lifestyle. Bowel management may be performed daily, or on alternate days, depending upon the individual's bowel pattern. The patient is encouraged to sit on a specially padded shower chair, so that bowel care can be performed over the toilet, followed by a shower. Sometimes this is not possible due to poor balance or preferred choice, and bowel management continues on the patient's bed.

Where possible, to promote independent care patients are taught manual evacuation if the bowel is flaccid, or suppositories are inserted and/or digital stimulation performed if they have a reflex bowel. If the patient is unable to carry out this activity, carers or district nurses are taught.

Sexuality

Following a spinal cord injury patients need to redefine sexuality and all that it encompasses. Nurses have to recognise when patients are ready to discuss sexuality, and respond appropriately as this need is not always verbalised in the early stages, and often manifests itself only in indirect questions or sexual innuendo. Discussion should be encouraged and should include dispelling myths, exploring the patient's new sexual status, looking at alternative methods, identifying practical problems; and advising on how to deal with them. Referral to medical staff, sexual health specialists and other agencies for further information and management, should be offered as appropriate.

Further reading

- Addison R, Smith M. *Digital rectal stimulation and manual removal of faeces. Guidance for nurses.* London: Royal College of Nursing, 2000
- Harrison P. *The first 48 hours.* London: Spinal Injuries Association, 2000
- Harrison P. *HDU/ICU. Managing spinal injury: critical care.* London: Spinal Injuries Association, 2000
- Leyson JFJ. *Sexual rehabilitation of the spinal cord injured patient.* Clifton, New Jersey: Humana Press, 1991
- Zejdlik CM. *Management of spinal cord injury*, 2nd edition. Boston: Jones and Bartlett Publishers, 1992

Box 8.15 Bowel management assessment

Consider
- Level of injury
- Pre-injury bowel pattern
- Diet/fluid intake
- What previously helped defaecation
- Hand function
- Balance/brace
- Psychological state

Box 8.16 Aims of bowel management

- Achieve regular bowel emptying by production of a formed stool at a chosen time and place
- Avoid leaks or unplanned emptying
- Avoid constipation and other complications
- Try to complete bowel care in 30–60 minutes
- Be as practical as possible

Box 8.17 Sexuality

- Acknowledge the need to discuss sexuality
- Redefine sexuality
- Dispel myths
- Explore opportunity and alternatives
- Advice to overcome practical difficulties

9   Physiotherapy

Trudy Ward, David Grundy

Physiotherapy assessment and treatment should be carried out as soon as possible after injury. During the early acute stage, care of the chest and paralysed limbs is of prime importance. Chest complications may occur as a result of the accident—for example, from inhaling water during diving incidents, from local complications such as fractured ribs, or from respiratory insufficiency caused by the level of the injury. Pre-existing lung disease may further complicate respiration.

Respiratory management

All patients receive prophylactic chest treatment, which includes deep breathing exercises, percussion and coughing, assisted if necessary. Careful monitoring is essential for tetraplegic patients as cord oedema may result in an ascending level of paralysis, further compromising respiration.

Patients with tetraplegia or high level paraplegia may have paralysed abdominal and intercostal muscles and will be unable to cough effectively. Assisted coughing will be necessary for effective lung clearance. Careful coordination and communication between physiotherapist and patient is vital for assisted coughing to be successful. Forced expiration may be achieved by the placement of the therapist's hands on either side of the lower ribs or on the upper abdomen and ribs, producing an upward and inward pressure as the patient attempts to cough. Two people may be needed to treat the patient with a wide chest or tenacious sputum.

Passive movements

All paralysed limbs are moved passively each day to maintain a full range of movement. Loss of sensation means that joints and soft tissues are vulnerable to overstretching, so great care must be taken not to cause trauma. Provided that stability of the bony injury is maintained, passive hip stretching with the patient in the lateral position, and strengthening of non-paralysed muscle groups, is encouraged.

Once the bony injury is stable patients will start sitting, preferably using a profiling bed, before getting up into a wheelchair. This is a gradual process because of the possibility of postural hypotension, which is most severe in patients with an injury above T6 and in the elderly.

Mobilisation into a wheelchair

Once a patient is in a wheelchair regular relief of pressure at the ischial, trochanteric, and sacral regions is essential to prevent the development of pressure sores in the absence of sensation. Patients must be taught to lift themselves to relieve pressure every 15 minutes. This must become a permanent habit. Paraplegic patients can usually do this without help by lifting on the wheels or arm rests of their wheelchairs. Tetraplegic patients should initially be provided with a cushion giving adequate pressure relief, but may in time be able to relieve pressure themselves.

Wheelchairs

Wheelchair design has been much influenced by technology. Lightweight wheelchairs are more aesthetically acceptable,

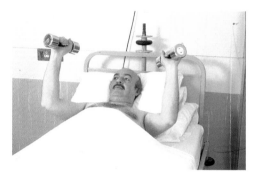

Figure 9.1 Patient with incomplete paraplegia using arm weights. Bilateral arm strengthening exercises must be done in supine position to maintain vertebral alignment.

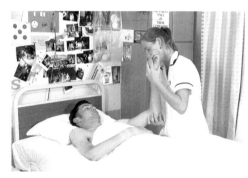

Figure 9.2 Passive movements to a patient's arm. Good support must be given to the paralysed joints and a full range of movement achieved.

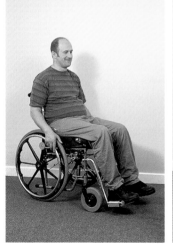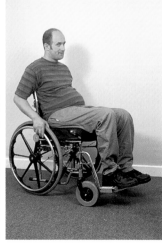

Figure 9.3 Left: patient correctly seated in wheelchair—erect and well back in the chair; footplates are level and adjusted to allow thighs to be fully supported on wheelchair cushion and for weight to be evenly distributed. Right: patient seated incorrectly—"slumped" and with poor trunk posture. Footplates are too high so there is excessive pressure on the sacrum—a potential pressure problem.

considerably easier to use, and often adjustable to the individual user's requirements. An appropriate wheelchair should be ordered once an assessment of the patient's ongoing needs has been made.

Rehabilitation

Physical rehabilitation includes the following:

- Familiarity with the wheelchair. The patient has to be taught how to propel the chair, operate the brakes, remove the footplates and armrests, and fold and transport the wheelchair. Basic skills include pushing on level and sloping ground and turning the chair.
- Relearning the ability to balance. The length of time this takes will depend on the degree of loss of proprioception and on trunk control.
- Strengthening non-paralysed muscles.
- Learning to transfer from wheelchair to bed, toilet, bath, floor, easy chair, and car. Teaching these skills is only possible once confidence in balance is achieved and there is sufficient strength in the arms and shoulder girdles. The degree of independence achieved by each patient will depend on factors such as the level of the lesion, the degree of spasticity, body size and weight, age, mental attitude, and the skill of the therapist. Patients who cannot transfer themselves will require help, and patient and helpers will spend time with therapists and nurses learning the techniques for pressure relief, dressing, transferring, and various wheelchair manoeuvres. The level of independence achievable by tetraplegic patients is shown on page 55 in chapter 10. Close cooperation between physiotherapists and occupational therapists helps patients to reach their full potential.
- Learning advanced wheelchair skills: backwheel balancing to allow easier manoeuvrability over rough ground and provide a means of negotiating kerbs; jumping the chair sideways for manoeuvrability in a limited space; and lifting the wheelchair in and out of a car unaided.

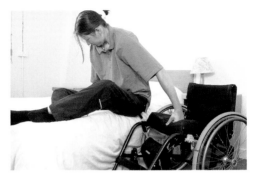

Figure 9.4 Patient with incomplete paraplegia below T6 transferring on to the bed. Having first lifted legs up on to the bed the patient then lifts rest of body horizontally from chair to bed. Hand position is important to achieve a safe lift, avoiding contact with wheel.

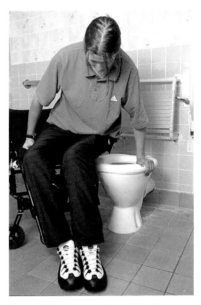

Figure 9.5 Patient with incomplete paraplegia below T6 transferring on to the toilet. Toilet seat must be well padded. Chair and legs must be carefully positioned to ensure a safe lift. Patient has to lift and rotate in one movement, so balance must be good and shoulder strength maximal.

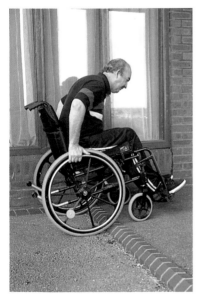

Figure 9.6 Patient going up kerb unaided. Patient must be able to balance on the rear wheels and travel forwards while maintaining this position and have enough strength to push chair up kerb.

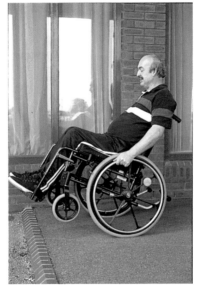

Figure 9.7 Patient coming down kerb unaided.

- Regular standing, may help to prevent contractures, reduce spasticity, and minimise osteoporosis. In patients subject to postural hypotension the vertical position must be assumed gradually, and patients may be helped by the use of an abdominal binder. For these patients the tilt table is used initially, progressing later, if appropriate, to an Oswestry standing frame or similar device.

Patients with low thoracic or lumbar lesions may be suitable for gait training using calipers and crutches, but success will depend on the patient's age, height, weight, degree of spasticity, and attitude. Orthotic devices such as the reciprocating gait orthosis (RGO), advanced reciprocating gait orthosis (ARGO), hip guidance orthosis (HGO), or Walkabout may be considered for patients including those unsuitable for traditional calipers and crutches. Instruction in the use of these devices requires specialist input and checks should be made on the patients and their orthoses at regular intervals.

Recreation

Sporting activities can be a valuable part of rehabilitation as they encourage balance, strength, and fitness, plus a sense of camaraderie and may well help patients reintegrate into society once they leave hospital. Archery, darts, snooker, table tennis, fencing, swimming, wheelchair basketball, and other athletic pursuits are all possible and are encouraged.

Incomplete lesions

Patients with incomplete lesions are a great challenge to physiotherapists as they present in various ways, which necessitates individual planning of treatment and continuing assessment. Patients with incomplete lesions may remain severely disabled despite neurological recovery. Spasticity may restrict the functional use of limbs despite apparently good isolated muscle power. The absence of proprioception or sensory appreciation will also hinder functional ability in the presence of otherwise adequate muscle power. Patients with a central cord lesion may be able to walk, but weakness in the arms may prevent them from dressing, feeding, or protecting themselves from falls. Recovery may well continue over several months, if not years, so careful review and referral to the patient's district physiotherapy department may be necessary to enable full functional potential to be achieved.

Children

Spinal cord injury in children is rare. The most important principles in the physical rehabilitation of the growing child with a spinal cord injury are preventing deformities, particularly scoliosis, and encouraging growth of the long bones. To achieve these aims the child requires careful bracing and full-length calipers to maintain an upright posture for as much of the day as possible. The child should be provided with a means of walking such as brace and calipers with crutches or rollator, a swivel walker, hip guidance orthosis, or reciprocating gait orthosis.

Sitting should be discouraged to prevent vertebral deformity. A wheelchair should be provided, however, to facilitate social activity both in and out of the home. Return to normal schooling is encouraged as soon as possible.

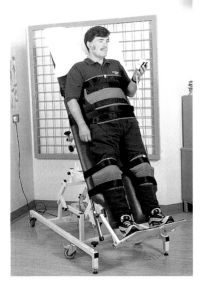

Figure 9.8 Tetraplegic patient standing on tilt table. Straps support patient's chest, lower trunk, and knees. Table is operated by therapist, the fully upright position being achieved gradually.

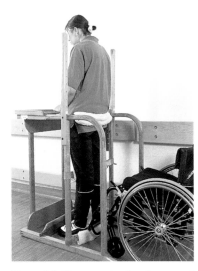

Figure 9.9 Oswestry standing frame enables paraplegic patient to stand by providing support through suitably placed padded straps at toes and heels, knees, and gluteal region. Uprights and two further straps supporting the trunk allow a tetraplegic patient to stand in the frame.

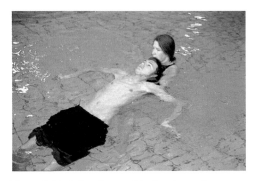

Figure 9.10 Swimming enables freedom of movement and independence, demonstrated here by a C6 tetraplegic.

Table 9.1 Gait expectations of patients with complete paraplegia: all patients should be totally independent with all transfers and chair manoeuvres both indoors and outdoors

Level of injury	Gait used	Descriptions
T1–T8	Gait—swing to with calipers and rollator May use crutches if spasticity is controlled	*Swing to gait* is the easiest type of gait to achieve but is slow and used only as an exercise. The patient puts the crutches a short distance in front of the feet and leans forward on to the crutches. He or she then pushes down with the shoulders, which lifts both legs together. The feet must land behind the crutches. It is a short, sharp lift. Prolonging the lift will make the feel go past the crutches and the patient will lose balance and fall.

T8–10	Swing to and swing through gait with full
	  length calipers and crutches
	Walking more likely to be an exercise
	  rather than fully functional
		Swing through gait is for speed and is the most functional for walking outside. However, it does expend a lot of energy. The patient places the crutches about 18 inches in front of the feet and leans forward on to the crutches; he or she then pushes the shoulder down, which raises both feet off the floor together. The lift must be maintained so that the feet are placed the same distance in front of the crutches as they started behind. As the feet touch the floor the patient must retract the shoulders to extend the hips and hence remain balanced.

T10–L2	Swing through and four point with calipers
	  and crutches
	Requires wheelchair for part of day—
	  walking may be fully functional	

L2–L4	Below knee calipers with crutches or sticks Wheelchair not required	*Four point gait* is the most difficult and requires excellent balance and strong shoulders and trunk. It is the nearest equivalent to a normal gait, but is very slow. The patient moves one crutch forward, transfers body weight on to the adjacent leg, and then moves the opposite leg forward by using latissimus dorsi to "hitch" the hip. The step must be short; if too large a step is taken the patient will fall, as he or she cannot recover balance.
L4–L5	May or may not require calipers Wheelchair not required May require sticks or other walking aid	

All the above depend on age, stature, amount and control of spasticity, any pre-existing medical condition, and the individual's motivation.

Young children have arms that are relatively short in relation to the trunk, so they should not attempt independent transfers. The child may therefore need to be readmitted and taught transfer skills at a later stage. Continued follow up is necessary throughout childhood, adolescence, and early adult life to ensure that adjustments are made to braces, calipers, and wheelchair to maintain good posture and correct growth.

Further reading

- Association of Swimming Therapy. *Swimming for people with disabilities.* London: A & C Black, 1992
- Bromley I. *Tetraplegia and paraplegia. A guide for physiotherapists,* 5th edition. Edinburgh: Churchill Livingstone, 1998
- Ward T. Spinal injuries. In: Pryor JA, Webber BA, eds. *Physiotherapy for respiratory and cardiac problems,* 2nd edition. Edinburgh: Churchill Livingstone, 1995, pp 429–38

10   Occupational therapy

Sue Cox Martin, David Grundy

The months in hospital after a spinal cord injury are an extremely difficult period for patients as they gradually adjust to what may be a lifetime of disability.

Occupational therapists are concerned with assisting patients to reach the maximum level of functional physical and psychological independence depending on the extent of the impairment, their home and social situation. Whalley Hammell suggests independence is not a physical state but more an attitude in which an individual takes on responsibility, solves problems, and establishes goals. Empowering an individual to make an informed choice about the way they choose to live their lives is not achieved in isolation, and therefore close working relationships with other professionals are essential.

The skills of the occupational therapist lie in assisting patients to overcome their difficulties, often by considering alternative methods and equipment to assist them with personal care, domestic tasks, and communication. The occupational therapist is also involved with advising people on home modifications, mobility including wheelchairs, driving and transport, returning to work, college or school, and the pursuit of leisure activities and hobbies.

Hand and upper limb management

Individual assessment of the hand and upper limb of tetraplegic patients is essential to maintain their hands in the optimum position for function.

Curtin describes the general acute management of patients with complete spinal cord injury, based on the level of lesion.

Hand management of patients with incomplete lesions needs close monitoring and if motor function improves activities are performed to enable the patient to achieve their maximum potential.

Tetraplegic patients with active wrist extensors should be encouraged to participate in activities to strengthen these muscles and to facilitate the use of their tenodesis grip. This occurs in the individual with a complete spinal cord lesion at C6 who is able to use active wrist extension to produce a grip between thumb and index fingers.

Some tetraplegic patients may require a variety of splints, such as those for writing and typing, wrist support splints, feeding straps, or pushing gloves, to enable them to carry out their daily activities. All splints are made individually for each patient by the therapist.

Some tetraplegic patients can benefit from reconstructive surgery to the hands or upper limbs, or both, but as surgery is not necessarily appropriate for all patients, careful preoperative assessment by a multidisciplinary team is vital. Staff in the spinal centre should carefully monitor postoperative care.

Home resettlement

Establishing early dialogue with the patient, the patient's family and friends is vital to enable the occupational therapist to be in a position to offer early advice and reassurance regarding living in the community. Early contact with the local social services is made as soon as possible after admission.

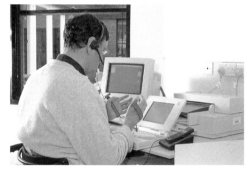

Figure 10.1 Technology enables a C6 complete tetraplegic writer to continue his work whilst undergoing rehabilitation.

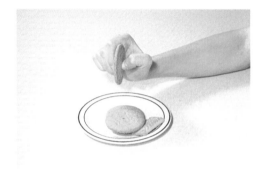

Figure 10.2 Active wrist extension in a C6 complete tetraplegic, enabling the patient to grip objects between thumb and index finger—a "tenodesis grip".

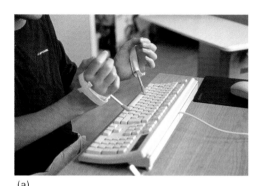

(a)

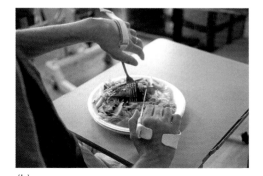

(b)

Figure 10.3 a) Using typing splints for a computer keyboard b) C6 tetraplegic eating meal with splints.

When an individual has a home to which they wish to return to, a joint visit may be carried out to give advice on its accessibility for overnight stays and for long-term resettlement. When an individual does not have a suitable home to return to alternatives are discussed, i.e. application to local authority for rehousing, purchase or rental of a new property.

An assessment visit involves a team from the spinal unit, including the occupational therapist and representatives from the patient's home area—usually the occupational therapist and social worker/care manager and the patient's family.

The visit begins the lengthy processes of planning for the patient's discharge and providing accessible accommodation. The timing usually means that the patient is unable to travel, and, although it is less than satisfactory for the patient to be absent, all ideas are discussed and decisions made with him or her and the family.

Recommendations are made to enable weekends to be spent away from hospital. Although facilities may be far from ideal, i.e. a hospital bed may have to be positioned in the living room, with no access to bathroom facilities, it is well recognised that time spent in the community provides the patient, family and friends with essential learning opportunities. Weekends away begin when the patient and family or friends feel confident to be away from the hospital. Enabling this to occur may involve the whole team in teaching techniques, procedures and instruction in the use of equipment to both patient and family.

Spending time away from the hospital may enable the patient, their family and friends to decide upon what plans they wish to make for long-term resettlement in the community.

If long-term alterations to a property are an option, grant aid towards the alterations may be available from the patient's local council and/or social services department, depending on the family's financial circumstances. The procedures involved in making alterations to a property require careful thought and planning and may take many months before completion.

As well as the availability of suitable accommodation, the organising of an appropriate care package may be necessary, which involves the whole team and may take time to organise.

In the event of completion of a patient's rehabilitation occurring before long-term accommodation is accessible or available, it may be necessary for alternative interim accommodation to be sought.

Activities of daily living

Once tetraplegic patients are out of bed and have started work on strengthening and balance, they begin to explore methods to relearn eating, drinking, washing, brushing their hair, cleaning their teeth, and shaving. Activities can be restricted due to the necessity of wearing a hard collar for the initial period of rehabilitation. These activities often entail the use of adapted tools or splints and straps made by the occupational therapist. The patient may need to relearn writing skills and may also explore the use of a computer, telephone, page-turner, and environmental control system.

As the patient becomes more confident and the wearing of a hard collar or brace all day is discontinued, he or she is able to progress to tasks involving bed mobility, in preparation for dressing, transfers, showering, and domestic activities. This can cover the whole range of domestic living and include being able to make a cup of tea, using a microwave, washing machine, vacuum cleaner or changing a duvet cover independently. Despite the patient's social situation they should be given the opportunity to relearn these activities.

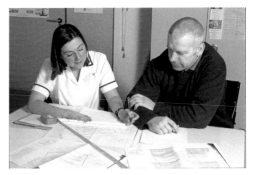

Figure 10.4 Discussing plans for an extension to the home with the occupational therapist.

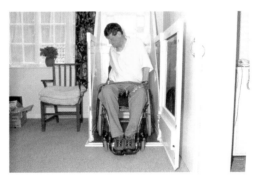

Figure 10.5 A complete C6 tetraplegic patient using a through-floor lift at home.

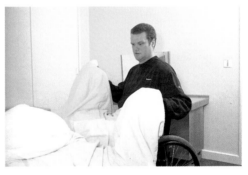

Figure 10.6 A T8 complete paraplegic changing a duvet cover independently.

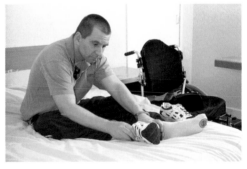

Figure 10.7 A T4 complete paraplegic dressing independently.

For patients who are unable to perform or assist in transfers the feasibility of being able to participate in hoisting may be pursued.

Communication

For tetraplegic patients unable to use their upper limbs functionally with standard communication systems, the role of the occupational therapist is to enable the patient to access alternative systems. Individual writing splints or mouthsticks may be made to enable those with limited writing skill to make a signature, which can be important to an individual for both business and personal correspondence. Alternative methods of being able to turn the pages of books, magazines and newspapers may be pursued.

Trial and selection of electrically powered equipment includes telephone, computer and assessment of environmental control systems, which can enable the individual to operate via a switch a range of functions, including television, video, intercom, computer, lights, radio, and accessing the telephone.

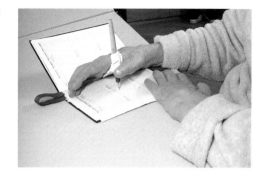

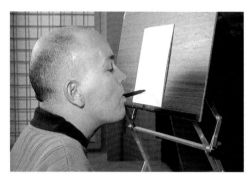

Figure 10.8 Communication. Top: a C6 complete tetraplegic using a writing splint. Bottom: a C4 complete tetraplegic using a mouthstick.

Box 10.1 Functional ability and anticipated level of independence of patients with complete tetraplegia

Complete lesion below C3:
- Diaphragm paralysed requires tracheostomy with permanent ventilation or diaphragm pacing
- Dependent on others for all personal and domestic care
- Able to use powered wheelchair with chin, head or breath control
- Able to use voice-activated computer
- Able to use electrically powered page-turner with switch
- Able to use environmental control equipment with switch, usually mouthpiece

Complete lesion below C4:
- Able to breathe independently using diaphragm
- Able to shrug shoulders
- Dependent on others for all personal and domestic care
- Able to use a powered wheelchair with chin control
- Able to use computer, either voice activated or using head switch or mouthstick
- Able to use environmental control equipment with mouthpiece as switch

Complete lesion below C5:
- Has shoulder flexion and abduction, elbow flexion and supination
- Able to participate in some aspects of personal and domestic care, i.e. eating, cleaning teeth using a wrist support and universal cuff
- Able to make signature using individually designed splint and wrist support
- Able to propel manual wheelchair short distances on level uncarpeted ground wearing pushing gloves and/or wrist supports
- Able to use powered wheelchair with joystick control for functional use
- May be able to assist with transfer from wheelchair onto level surfaces using a sliding board and an assistant
- Able to drive from wheelchair in an accessible vehicle
- Able to use environmental control equipment using a switch

Complete lesion below C6:
- Able to extend wrists

- Able to perform some aspects of personal and domestic care using a universal cuff
- Able to make a signature using an individually designed splint
- Able to dress upper half of body independently, but may require some assistance with dressing lower half of body
- Able to propel wheelchair, including slopes
- May be independent in bed, car, and shower chair transfers
- Able to drive an automatic car with hand controls

Complete lesion below C7:
- Full wrist movement and some hand function, but no finger flexion or fine hand movements
- Able to be independent in bed, car, shower chair, and toilet transfers
- May require assistance/equipment to assist with wheelchair to floor transfers
- Able to dress and undress independently
- Able to drive an automatic car with hand controls

Complete lesion below C8:
- All hand muscles except intrinsics preserved
- Wheelchair independent but may have difficulty going up and down kerbs
- Able to drive an automatic car with hand controls

Complete lesion below T1:
- Complete innervation of arms
- Wheelchair independent
- Able to drive an automatic car with hand controls

These expectations are general and depend upon the patient's age, physical proportions, physical stamina and agility, degree of spasticity and motivation. In incomplete spinal cord lesions, where there can be variable potential for neurological recovery, it may not be possible to predict functional outcome, which can lead to increased anxiety for the patient.

The level of independence achieved by children not only depends on their size and functional ability but the attitude of their parents. As the adult with a spinal cord lesion becomes older their ability to maintain their level of independence may diminish and require review.

Mobility

Wheelchairs

Whenever possible an individual is encouraged to propel his or her wheelchair as soon as they are able. Pushing gloves and/or wrist supports may be required.

As soon as is practicable liaison occurs between the spinal centre staff, the patient and the patient's local district wheelchair service. They are able to assess and provide wheelchairs from a range, which includes self-propelling, lightweight, indoor powered, indoor/outdoor powered and attendant-operated wheelchairs. Initially a patient may be issued with a basic wheelchair and reassessed once he or she is able to participate in choosing a long-term wheelchair. The occupational therapist should be able to guide the individual to trial and select a wheelchair with features that suit the patient's functional ability and lifestyle.

An extensive range of wheelchairs is available commercially, including those that tilt in space and enable standing, and outdoor powered wheelchairs.

Driving and vehicles

Several centres specialise in assessing an individual prior to returning to driving and give advice on the trial and selection of controls that suit an individual's functional ability. The assessment also includes advice on methods of storage of the wheelchair in the vehicle. For individuals who wish to remain in their wheelchair whilst travelling, either as a driver or a passenger, the choice of wheelchair must be matched with the choice of vehicle and the individual's size.

Leisure

Constructive use of leisure time is vital to maintain self-esteem and self-confidence. Some previous activities and interests can be continued, with a little thought and suitable adjustment. There are many national groups and organisations with facilities to support individuals to pursue their hobbies, sporting interests, travel and holidays, and access to the internet has widened the range of information available.

Work

Work is of varying importance to patients, but some will see it as giving a sense of purpose to their life and will want to return to their former occupation if at all possible. Early contact with the patient's employer to discuss the feasibility of eventual return to his or her previous job is important. If the degree of a patient's disability precludes this, some employers are sympathetic and flexible and will offer a job that will be possible from a wheelchair.

As a result of their spinal cord injury, some people use the opportunity to take stock of their lives and retrain or enter further education. Some people choose not to return to paid employment but seek occupation in the voluntary sector. Many patients find life outside hospital difficult enough initially, however, without the added responsibility of a job, and in these circumstances a period of adjustment at home is advisable before they return to work. When such patients feel ready to

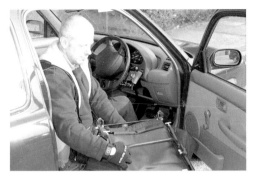

Figure 10.9 A T12 paraplegic transferring into a car and lifting the wheelchair into the passenger seat.

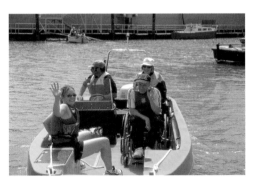

Figure 10.10 Leisure.

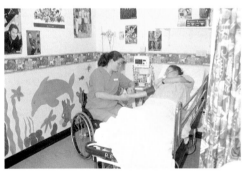

Figure 10.11 A T5 paraplegic nurse treating a patient in the emergency department.

consider some alternative employment they can contact their local employment service, which may be able to offer practical advice and financial support.

If a patient is planning to return to his or her previous employer, school, or college, the occupational therapist is able to assess the suitability of the premises for wheelchair accessibility and make recommendations on the facilities which would be necessary. The advance of information technology has increased employment opportunities for patients of all levels of lesion who choose to return to work.

Further reading

- Curtin M. Development of a tetraplegic hand assessment and splinting protocol. *Paraplegia* 1994;**32**:159–69
- Whalley Hammell K. *Spinal cord injury rehabilitation.* London: Chapman and Hall 1995

11   Social needs of patient and family

Julia Ingram, David Grundy

The aim of successful rehabilitation is to enable the patient to live as satisfactory and fulfilling a life as possible. This will mean different choices and decisions for each individual depending on the degree of disability, the family and social environment, and preferred lifestyle.

The vast majority of patients want to live in their own homes and not in residential care, and very severely disabled people achieve this successfully. Many will live as part of a family or, increasingly, choose to live independently with support from community services. Caring for People (Cm 849, 1989) recognised this, and in April 1993 the legislation was enacted, facilitating provision of care in the community, and for the first time the needs of carers were specifically mentioned. The Independent Living Fund (1993) has made payments to people with severe disabilities to enable them to purchase care to supplement that provided by family and local health and social services. The introduction of Direct Payments provides opportunities for people to take control of their local authority funded packages. Resource shortfalls, however, are causing increasing difficulties.

For most people spinal cord injury demands changes in almost every aspect of life—personal relationships, the physical structure of the home, work and education, social and leisure pursuits, and financial management. Consequently, exhaustive and careful planning by the spinal unit staff and staff responsible for community services, in conjunction with the patient and family, is essential. Because of the complexities and scale of what is required, this planning should start as soon after injury as possible. Planning before discharge is only the start of a lifelong, probably fluctuating, need for services. In providing these, the social and emotional wellbeing of the person and family must be considered along with physical health. Physical health supports and is supported by a satisfactory lifestyle.

Table 11.1 Where patients are living: figures based on acute injury discharges from The Duke of Cornwall Spinal Treatment Centre 1998–99

Where patients are living	%
Living with relatives after discharge	29
Living independently or with partner on discharge	57
Required interim residential care on discharge	7
Transferred to other hospital	7

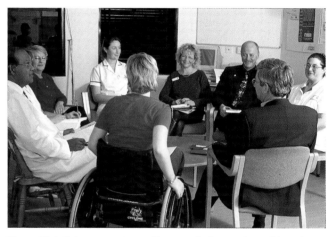

Figure 11.1 Primary care team discusses discharge plans with patient and family.

Changed relationships

The onset of severe disability can have profound effects, not necessarily damaging, on existing personal relationships and on the formation of new relationships. Disability will change the roles people have in a relationship: for instance, some may find that they have to manage the family's financial and business affairs for the first time, or others may have to undertake extra household tasks. The able-bodied person—husband, wife, partner, son, daughter or parent—may have to provide intimate personal care. The 1995 Carers Act makes it possible for carers to have assessments of their own needs if the person they care for has an assessment under the NHS and Community Care Act 1990. Further legislation aims to make these assessments available to carers in their own right, through the Carers and Disabled Childrens Act 2000.

The workload of everyone concerned is likely to be much greater. For many couples an active and satisfying sexual relationship will be possible, but it will be different. These changes, in addition to the feelings engendered by loss of function and its actual cause, are likely to have major repercussions.

Many spinal cord injuries happen to late adolescents or young adults at the stage when they are beginning to form relationships

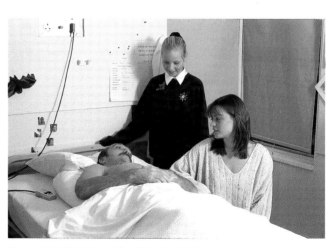

Figure 11.2 Patient and family in hospital.

and establish independence from parents, and they may be very concerned about their ability to do so. It takes time and the realisation that people do think that they are still worthwhile before necessary self-esteem can return. These adjustments are likely to take place after discharge from hospital because then the issues become clearer. Many people find that the initial period after discharge can be very stressful.

Work is of varying importance to patients, but most will see it as giving a sense of purpose to their life and crucial to their self-esteem, and will want to return to their former occupation if at all possible. Early contact with the patient's employer to discuss the feasibility of eventual return to his or her previous job is important. If the degree of a patient's disability precludes this, some employers are sympathetic and flexible and will offer a job that will be possible from a wheelchair. However, many patients initially find life outside hospital difficult enough, having to cope with their disability and adjust to living again in the community, without having the added responsibility of a job. In these circumstances a period of adjustment at home is advisable before they return to work, as it may be two or three years or longer before a patient is psychologically rehabilitated.

If patients are keen to return to their previous job, school, or college, the occupational therapist should assess the suitability of the premises for wheelchair accessibility. Recommendations are then made to the placement, assessment, and counselling team (PACT) or local education authority, if alterations to the buildings or the installation of specialised equipment are needed to make them suitable for the patient.

When such patients feel ready to consider some alternative employment they can contact their local disability employment adviser.

If patients are considering returning to work, time spent in a rehabilitation workshop can be helpful. In this environment they should be able to test their aptitude for activities such as carpentry, engineering, electronics and computer work, build up their strength, concentration, and stamina, and have a clearer idea of their employment capabilities.

Good community support, including practical help with the tasks of caring, and also the imaginative provision of resources to enable the person and carers to participate in normal community activities, are likely to help the process. Tired people who have limited social satisfactions will find it more difficult to make the necessary adjustments.

Counselling can be a valuable source of help in making these adjustments. Studies indicate that people with spinal cord injuries are not as psychologically distressed or depressed by their injury as able-bodied people, including experienced staff, imagine. Many people with spinal cord injury do lead active fulfilling lives, though this may take time to achieve.

Finance

Adequate finance is a major factor in determining successful rehabilitation, but many severely disabled people are living in poverty.

Not only do patients and their families have to cope with all the stresses of injury; they may have to live on a severely reduced income which cannot support their existing lifestyle. It is also more expensive to live as a disabled person. Disability Living Allowance, or Attendance Allowance for over 65 year olds, provides some help with the more obvious costs, but no provision exists for tasks such as decorating, repairs, and gardening, which the disabled person may no longer be able to perform.

Even if the person receives financial compensation this may take several years to be granted, and though interim payments

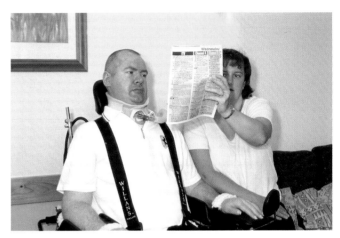

Figure 11.3 Ventilator-dependent tetraplegic with carer.

Box 11.1 Finance—major factor in determining successful rehabilitation

- Welfare benefits often complex
- Disabled people often receive less than their entitlement
- Disabled people need advice on benefits due to them

Box 11.2 Benefits commonly available to disabled people

Benefits to assist with disability:
- Disability Living Allowance (DS 704)
- Attendance Allowance (if over 65 years of age) (DS 702)
- Disabled Person's Tax Credit (information available from the Inland Revenue)
- Industrial Disablement Benefit (DB1)
- NHS Charges and Optical Voucher Values (HC12)
- Help with Health Costs (HC11)

Income maintenance benefits:
- Statutory Sick Pay (for 28 weeks) (information available from the Inland Revenue) if in employment and not self employed

or
- Incapacity Benefit (IB1+IB203) up to 28 weeks if self-employed or unemployed. After 28 weeks for all groups. Dependent on sufficient National Insurance contributions (SD2). If 16–20, or under 25 and in full time education, contributions discounted

If *not* enough contributions
- Income Support (IS20) means tested (SD2)
- Severe Disablement Allowance (if eligible) (SD3) if claimed before April 2001. Discounted since then for new applicants

Income Support will "top up" any of the above if income is below the assessed needs level.

- War Disablement Pension (WPA—leaflet—1)
- Housing Benefit and Council Tax Benefit (administered by district councils) (RR2)
- Invalid Care Allowance (SD4) (paid to some carers)
- Working Families Tax Credit (information available from the Inland Revenue)

(DSS leaflet numbers are given in parentheses)

can be made, in some circumstances they are not always available at the time of discharge from hospital, when there is likely to be major expenditure on either moving or adapting the present house.

Because of the interruption in, or possible loss of, earning capacity many people will be dependent for long periods on welfare benefits administered by the Department of Social Security. These are complex, and various studies have shown that many disabled people are receiving less than their entitlement, sometimes by quite substantial amounts. It is therefore important for those working with disabled people to be aware that they may be underclaiming benefits and to advise them accordingly.

Adapting homes

Most houses are unsuitable for wheelchairs unless adapted. Disabled Facilities Grants may be available to assist with the cost, but for many people help is limited because mortgage repayments are not taken into account in the financial assessment. Housing presents a continuing problem because, though patients may return to an adapted house or be rehoused from hospital, they may well want to change house in the future, especially as spinal cord injuries typically occur in young people who would normally move house several times. A disabled person may have difficulty in finding a suitable house, and there can be time restrictions on further provision of grants for adaptations. There are also mandatory and discretionary limitations on grants which may be made available to assist in the adaptation of a property. Many people find the discrepancy between local authorities in their interpretation of the legislation around this frustrating. Many cannot afford to buy a house and will depend on council housing, housing association property, or privately rented property, all of which are in short supply. Consequently, any move can be difficult to achieve and has to be planned well ahead. The services of community occupational therapists, housing departments, and social workers may be required.

A considerable number of statutory services are concerned with providing services for disabled people. Voluntary organisations also provide important resources. They can act as pressure and self-help groups, and organisations of disabled people have the knowledge and understanding born of personal experience. There are many such organisations, of which the Spinal Injuries Association is particularly relevant.

To mobilise and coordinate these services, which often vary in what they can provide in different geographical areas, is a major undertaking. Too often disabled people fail to receive a service that would be of benefit or they may feel overwhelmed and not in control of their own lives, with consequent damage to morale and health. Disabled people and their families should have access to full information about the services available and be enabled to make their own decisions about what they need. The 1998 White Paper Modernising Social Services sets out government objectives for more partnership working, joint funding and uniformity of charging policies across local authorities which should make services more accessible to patients and with greater parity.

Table 11.2 Adapting homes—where patients go: figures based on acute injury discharges from The Duke of Cornwall Spinal Treatment Centre 1998–99

Where patients go	%
Able to return to own home with adaptations	55
Had to move to live with relatives	11
Required rehousing provided by District Council or Housing Association	29
Required rehousing, patient or family bought property	5

Box 11.3 Typical adaptations funded either privately or in part by a Disabled Facilities Grant

- Ramped access to external doors
- Widening of internal doors
- Level access parking, with carport/garage
- Level access shower
- Toilet with access for shower chair
- Accessible light switches, sockets, door locks
- Accessible kitchen and facilities
- Patio area in the garden
- Thermostatically controlled heating system
- Through-floor lift or stair lift
- Internal ramps

Table 11.3 Employment—what patients do: figures based on acute injury discharges from The Duke of Cornwall Spinal Treatment Centre 1998–99

Employment—what patients do	%
In work or job left open	30
In education or training	10
No employment on discharge, but previously employed	38
No employment on discharge—not employed when admitted	22

Box 11.4 Information and advice on benefits

- Department of Social Security (local office or DSS) Benefit Enquiry Line. Tel: 0800 882200
- Citizens Advice Bureau
- DIAL (Disabled Information Advice Line) (Name of town)—A voluntary organisation operating in some areas
- Disability Rights Handbook (Price £11.50 post free); published annually by the Disability Alliance Educational & Research Association, Universal House, 88–94 Wentworth Street, London E1 7SA. Tel: 020 77247 8776.
- Spinal Injuries Association—76 St James's Lane, London N10 3DF. Tel: 020 8444 2121 or 0800 980 0501. www.spinal.co.uk. email: sia@spinal.co.uk

12   Transfer of care from hospital to community

Rachel Stowell, Wendy Pickard, David Grundy

Discharge from hospital is a complicated process for both paraplegic and tetraplegic patients. Physical care is a major concern, and here the difference between levels of injury is profound. People with paraplegia usually become self caring; those with low tetraplegia, especially if young, may also achieve independence, but those with high tetraplegia may require help with their physical needs.

Achievement of good care depends largely on educating the patients, their families, and the community staff. Patients should be expert at understanding and, as far as possible, caring for their own bodies. They need to be able to recognise potential problems and either deal with them themselves or know where to seek advice. Much time is spent in teaching the importance of good skin, bladder and bowel care, as long-term problems in these areas are common.

Education of patients

Skin care

Patients are taught how to use a mirror to check their pressure areas regularly, the stages of development of pressure sores, and what to do should a pressure mark occur. Wheelchairs and cushions are best assessed in a pressure clinic. If patients cannot lift themselves in their chair they need a cushion that allows them to sit in their wheelchair all day without resulting in a red mark on their skin. Weight, height, the degree of sensation and mobility, age, posture, motivation, and the quality of the skin all affect the type of cushion needed. All wheelchair cushions have a limited life and need regular checking to provide a reliable degree of assistance in prevention of sores.

Clothes made of natural fibres are preferable because many patients sweat excessively; clothing should not be tight otherwise there is risk of skin damage resulting in pressure sores. It should also be noted that hard seams and pockets which cross over the ischial tuberosities, trochanters, or coccyx may cause pressure marks on the skin. It is recommended that shoes should generally be one size larger than previously worn because of a tendency of the feet to swell during the day.

The choice of a suitable mattress is also important. Many pressure-relieving mattresses are now available, so all patients should be able to sleep for at least eight hours without being turned, and without resulting in a red mark on their skin. The patient should be assessed individually to ascertain the appropriate mattress for their long-term needs. Patients are encouraged to contact the pressure clinic for information and advice regarding any aspect of their care. In addition, the community liaison staff while visiting the patient in the community are able to reinforce educational aspects.

Bladder care

Patients are taught the most effective method of bladder emptying (see chapter 7). Although men with high tetraplegia can often tap over the bladder to induce a detrusor contraction, they may require help to apply a sheath and to fit a leg bag. In women with high tetraplegia the bladder is often

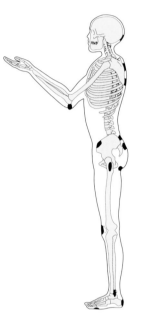

Box 12.1 People need to develop skills in:
• Understanding and caring for their own bodies
• Recognising potential problems
• Dealing with problems or learning where to go for advice

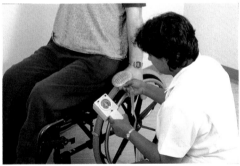

Figure 12.1 Top: areas of skin most at risk of effects of pressure. Bottom: skin pressure elevator to measure the pressure between the skin and supporting surface.

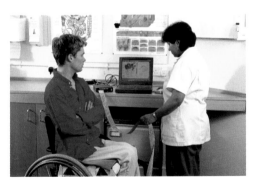

Figure 12.2 Force sensing array: pressure mapping can be used to assess pressure distribution, which helps to prevent skin breakdown.

best managed by a suprapubic catheter. It is best to avoid long-term urethral catheters as these may damage the bladder neck and urethra. Patients whose bladder emptying method involves an indwelling catheter are taught to regularly use a catheter valve (which can be opened and closed), to maintain bladder volume and compliance. Intermittent clean self-catheterisation is the preferred method for most women and men with paraplegia and some with low tetraplegia. It is particularly successful in patients with an acontractile bladder.

Long-term bladder management

Urinary tract infections are common but may be reduced by adequate hydration and often by urinary acidification. In general antibiotics are given only when an infection causes systemic symptoms. If recurrent urinary tract infections occur the patient should be investigated for underlying causes such as stones in the urinary tract or poor bladder emptying. Various surgical interventions are available in selected patients (see chapter 7).

Bowel care

Patients with tetraplegia and paraplegia who have an upper motor neurone cord lesion generally have reflex bowel activity, and evacuation can usually be produced by inserting glycerine suppositories or by anal digital stimulation, or both. Patients with high tetraplegia generally have poor balance and have to be hoisted on to a padded shower chair which can be wheeled over a toilet. This is more acceptable than being hoisted directly on to a toilet, which is generally less stable. In some circumstances bowel evacuation may need to take place on the bed with the patient in the left lateral position.

Patients with low paraplegia and a lower motor neurone cord lesion generally have a flaccid bowel, so will need to evacuate their bowel manually or by straining using the abdominal muscles, or by a combination of the two methods. Patients who carry out manual evacuation are advised to keep their stools slightly constipated to ease removal. They should be able to transfer themselves onto a toilet, and the seat should be padded to prevent pressure sores from developing due to prolonged sitting. In practice most patients evacuate their bowels daily or on alternate days. When possible, the timing and frequency of bowel evacuation should be made to fit in with the person's lifestyle. Help can be requested from the district nurse. Patients are advised to maintain their bowel regime and to avoid strong oral and rectal stimulant laxatives and enemas. Further educational principles are described in chapter 8 on nursing.

Long-term bowel management

A change in diet or lifestyle can affect bowel management, and patients are advised to change only one aspect of their bowel care at a time to minimise potential problems. Long-term options which can address chronic bowel management problems include colonic irrigation via the rectum, or through an abdominal stoma (an antegrade colonic enema), or a stoma, such as a colostomy.

Autonomic dysreflexia

Autonomic dysreflexia is commonly associated with bladder or bowel problems, particularly overdistension. By the time of discharge from hospital, patients should be fully aware of the signs and symptoms of autonomic dysreflexia and be able to direct people to help find and remove the cause (see chapter 6).

Box 12.2 Long-term bladder management

- Intermittent self-catheterisation is preferred method for those with acontractile bladders
- Condom sheath drainage in contractile bladders
- If indwelling catheter, suprapubic catheter is preferable to urethral catheter, to avoid urethral damage. Use catheter valve to maintain bladder compliance and capacity

---

Box 12.3 Urinary tract infections

- Treat with antibiotics only if systemic symptoms present
- Adequate hydration and urinary acidification
- Investigate recurrent infections

Box 12.4 Bowel

- Upper motor neurone cord lesion ⟶ reflex emptying—responds to suppositories and anal digital stimulation
- Lower motor neurone cord lesion ⟶ flaccid bowel with emptying by manual evacuation

---

Box 12.5 Long-term bowel management

- Daily or on alternate days
- Maintain consistent bowel regime
- Avoid strong laxatives and enemas
- Should fit in with patient's lifestyle
- Change in diet or lifestyle can affect bowel management
- Only change one aspect of bowel care at a time, to minimise potential problems

---

Box 12.6 Autonomic dysreflexia

High lesion patients must:
- be aware of the signs and symptoms
- be able to direct care.

Nutrition

Patients with spinal cord injury, particularly those with high lesions, are often unable to exercise adequately and are prone to excessive weight gain, which can further limit their mobility and independence. In the long term, most patients tend to be constipated and will benefit from dietary re-education. A diet of good nutritional standard but with a controlled calorific content is important. Care needs to be taken in changing the diet if constipation, or more seriously diarrhoea with a risk of bowel accidents, is to be avoided.

> **Box 12.7 Nutrition**
> - Prone to excessive weight gain
> - Diet of good nutritional standard, to include 5 servings of fruit and vegetables per day
> - Change of diet affects bowel management

Teaching the family and community staff

When patients are discharged from hospital they should be thoroughly responsible for their own care. If the patient wishes, family members are given individual instruction on how to help in their care and have the opportunity to attend a study day about all aspects of spinal cord injury. If it is envisaged that the patient will require help in the community, district nurses and carers are invited to the spinal unit to work with the primary care teams, thereby enabling them to learn specific aspects of care for their prospective patients. The community staff can also be invited to attend study days which include the subjects of pressure sore prevention, bladder and bowel management, activities of daily living, long-term aspects of spinal cord injury, and psychological support. Most community staff welcome the opportunity to visit the spinal unit as spinal cord injury is not very common.

The community liaison staff based at the spinal unit will also visit community staff to give support and advice.

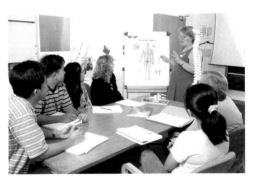

Figure 12.3 Formal teaching session.

Preparation for discharge from hospital

Providers of care

Patients with high tetraplegia require a substantial amount of care, which will be given by other people. Traditionally this care has been provided by the patient's family. The family should not be expected to take responsibility for the delivery of care, however, especially as it will be required for many years, and they may already have work commitments that are financially necessary. Usually, people with a high level of disability wish to maintain their independence as much as possible and so choose to live independently, therefore it is essential that they have help to do this. The patient may require the services of district nurses and local care agencies. With financial support the patient may be able to employ their own care such as a live-in carer or personal assistant.

Independent living becomes an achievable goal for the patient with the utilisation of these support services. If help and support are not given when the patient goes home from hospital this can increase pressure on the family unit and lead to the breakdown of relationships. Even if the family members are not providing the physical care it is important that they have their own space and time otherwise resentment can occur along with physical and emotional exhaustion.

> **Box 12.8 Providers of care**
> - District nurses
> - Care assistants
> - Resident carers/personal assistants:
>   Privately employed
>   Employed by disabled person using state benefits
> - Family

Planning for discharge home

Preparation for discharge home should start soon after the patient is admitted to a spinal unit. Many patients with a spinal cord injury are young and were already making decisions about their future. It is very difficult for them to make major choices

> **Box 12.9 Planning for discharge home**
> - Commence plans for discharge as early as possible
> - Major decisions to make regarding future plans
> - May need temporary solution
> - Flexible thinking for planning discharge

of where to live and with whom and to decide who may be able to help them with their care. It is sometimes necessary to have a temporary solution, and when they have had more time to adjust to their injury a more permanent solution can be found. It is therefore essential that this initial decision should allow a certain amount of flexibility.

Planning for independent living

Many patients with tetraplegia choose to live independently, and initially statutory care facilities in the patient's home may be used. These services may not be able to meet fully the care needs of someone with a high level of injury so they may need to be supplemented. Many people will prefer to employ a personal assistant to live in to help with personal care and daily living activities. This allows people to take control of their lives but requires them to develop skills in interviewing, financial management, and teaching. When financial compensation for the injury is not available staff from the spinal unit contact the patient's local social services and health care trusts for financial support through community care assessment, the Independent Living Fund (ILF), and direct payment scheme. Initially, patients choosing this option often require additional support from the spinal unit for advice in relation to, for instance, advertising for carers and interviewing. Patients quickly become totally responsible for their own care on leaving the spinal unit.

Planning for interim care

When their homes have not been adapted for wheelchair use before the patients' discharge from the spinal unit, interim care may be necessary and can help to act as a bridge between the protection of a spinal injuries unit and the reality of everyday living with a disability.

Easing transfer from hospital to community

The support of the district nursing service is invaluable in easing the transfer from the spinal unit to the community. Before discharge patients will have some weekends at home. Difficulties experienced by them and their families can be discussed with the district nurse and care agency, who can assess the situation and contact the spinal unit if advice is required. The families are often reassured to know that there is an effective link between the spinal unit and the community. To maintain this link the initial discharge plan may require a district nurse each morning to provide personal care with help from a care assistant.

The early weeks at home

The early weeks after discharge can be both physically and emotionally exhausting for all concerned. The patients are faced with the harsh reality of everyday living. However well a patient's community care is planned, problems may still arise. For this reason all patients are visited by the community liaison staff from the spinal unit usually within 6–8 weeks of discharge and at other times as required at the request of the patient, family, carers, district nurse, or general practitioner. Community liaison staff will meet with community staff and visit patients together to educate and further ease the transfer of care from the spinal unit to home.

Aim for independent living

To become totally responsible for their own care on discharge from spinal unit

Box 12.10 Skills required for independent living

- Interviewing, employing and training staff
- Managing personal finances
- Effective communication skills—assertiveness
 —telephone skills

Box 12.11 Planning for interim care

Acts as a bridge between:
- protection of a spinal injuries unit
- reality of everyday living with a disability

Box 12.12 Transfer from hospital to community eased by:

- Single and joint visits from:
 District nurse (once a day initially)
 Care assistant
 Community liaison staff from spinal unit (within 6–8 weeks after discharge from hospital, thereafter on request)

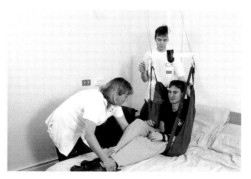

Figure 12.4 Patient in a hoist.

Travel and holidays

When considering travelling and holidays it is important that this is well planned to ensure there is no risk to the patient's health. There are a few specific areas that will need to be addressed.

Skin care

If there is some uncertainty about the condition of the mattress the patient will be sleeping on while away from home, it is wise for the patient to take an overlay mattress in the luggage.

Bladder care

If the patient normally manages his/her bladder by intermittent self-catheterisation and is going on a long journey, such as a long flight, it may be more practicable to have an indwelling urethral catheter for the duration of the flight, due to difficult access to toilet facilities. If the patient is travelling to a hot country fluid intake should be increased and catheters adjusted accordingly.

Bowel care

Different food, particularly spicy dishes, may affect a patient's bowel habit. Patients are advised to adjust their bowel regime accordingly, and are taught how to carry out bowel care on a bed, should toilets be inaccessible.

Cushions

When travelling on a plane, patients are advised to keep their cushions with them and not to allow them to be stored in the hold with the wheelchair, as they can easily get lost. It may be necessary for patients to sit on their cushions whilst on a plane to aid pressure relief, particularly on long journeys.

Patients should seek advice from their spinal unit, or an association such as the Spinal Injuries Association, prior to travelling.

Follow-up

Patients are followed up as outpatients by their spinal unit. This consists of regular outpatient appointments, which normally include a yearly renal ultrasound and abdominal *x* ray. During these appointments it is important that the patient has access to a multidisciplinary team who can provide ongoing assessment of the patient's health care needs, and minimise the incidence of potential problems. It is also important that patients have access to telephone advice and community visits from a spinal unit, and that they are aware of information resources available to them, such as the Spinal Injuries Association.

Further reading

- Addison R, Smith M. *Digital rectal stimulation and manual removal of faeces. Guidance for nurses.* London: Royal College of Nursing, 2000
- Fowler CJ, ed. *Neurology of bladder, bowel and sexual dysfunction.* Oxford: Butterworth Heinemann, 1999
- *Moving 'further' forward—the guide to living with spinal cord injury.* London: Spinal Injuries Association, 1999. [Provides a wealth of information for spinal cord injured patients and their carers]

Box 12.13 Travel and holidays

- Plan well ahead
- Ascertain condition of mattress—use an overlay
- Air flights—indwelling urethral catheter may be needed
    —keep wheelchair cushion during flight and sit on it if possible
- Increase fluid intake in hot climates
- Spicy food may affect bowel management
- Bowel care may need to be carried out on a bed
- Seek advice from the spinal unit prior to travelling abroad

Box 12.14 Follow-up

- Regular outpatient clinic appointments
- Regular renal ultrasound and abdominal *x* ray
- Access to a multidisciplinary team
- Telephone support and advice from spinal unit
- Information resources—Spinal Injuries Association

13 Later management and complications—I

David Grundy, Anthony Tromans, Firas Jamil

Late spinal instability and spinal deformity

Clinicians should be alert to the possibility of late spinal instability in patients who have sustained spinal trauma. Pain, increasing deformity and, less frequently, the appearance of a new neurological deficit, are the usual manifestations.

Preventing spinal deformity is extremely important, particularly as correcting an established deformity may be difficult and potentially hazardous if major surgery is necessary. It is therefore important to diagnose and treat spinal instability at an early stage. Patients who have sustained flexion or flexion-distraction injuries to the spine are most at risk of spinal instability, due to the high incidence of posterior spinal column and ligamentous damage. The most important factors contributing to missed instability are the presence of multiple injuries, in particular head injury, the occurrence of spinal injuries at more than one level, and spinal cord injury without radiological abnormality (SCIWORA) which can represent a ligamentous injury.

The most important factors predisposing to spinal deformity are the nature of the original bony or ligamentous injury, age at injury and the level and completeness of the cord lesion. The growing child is most at risk of developing a major spinal deformity, usually a scoliosis. The higher the neurological level and the more complete the lesion, the greater the tendency to spinal deformity.

Inadequate early treatment of the bony injury or inappropriate surgical exploration by laminectomy without stabilisation and fusion may also lead to late deformity. Inadequate postural management, particularly in seating, with muscle imbalance, may lead to an excessive lumbar lordosis with an anterior pelvic tilt. Conversely a severe lumbar kyphosis with the patient sitting on the sacrum is often associated with the development of a long paralytic scoliosis. Lower limb deformities may also affect the spine—for instance, flexion contractures of the hips cause pelvic obliquity and excessive lumbar lordosis, and if the deformity is asymmetrical scoliosis will result. An optimum posture will reduce the risk of pressure sores.

In children spinal bracing is required until vertebral growth is completed, and until then periods of sitting should be limited. An erect frame such as a swivel walker and a prone trolley to limit sitting in a wheelchair are helpful, particularly in the very young. In adults with thoracolumbar injury bracing is often advisable even if internal fixation has been performed. High thoracic spinal deformity severe enough to require surgical correction requires careful preoperative assessment, respiratory complications being a particular hazard of the operation.

In patients with incomplete neurological lesions and a severe deformity, the risk of developing a secondary myelopathy if treated conservatively has to be weighed against the considerable risk of major surgery, requiring a combined anterior and posterior approach.

Pathological fractures

Although internal fixation of limb fractures sustained at the time of the spinal cord injury may often be indicated,

Box 13.1 Predisposing factors

- Nature of original bony injury
- Age at injury
- Level of lesion
- Completeness of lesion
- Inadequate treatment of bony injury
- Laminectomy without stabilisation and fusion
- Gross leg deformities

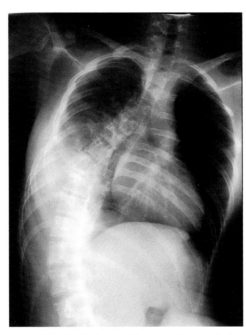

Figure 13.1 Scoliosis complicating a T4 paraplegia in a 16-year-old female patient.

Box 13.2 Spinal deformity may:

- Predispose to pressure sores due to pelvic obliquity and excessive lumbar lordosis
- Result in decreased lung compliance and potential respiratory embarrassment

Box 13.3 Prime objective of management of spinal deformity is to prevent progression by:

- Seating and positioning
- Correction of posture
- Bracing
- Surgery in selected cases

particularly to assist nursing, the emphasis later is on a more conservative approach. After injury to the spinal cord, bones in the paralysed limbs become osteoporotic, and pathological fractures may occur with minimal or even no obvious trauma. A common injury is a supracondylar fracture of the femur caused by the patient falling out of the wheelchair on to his or her knees. Violent spasticity of the hip flexors, particularly if the leg rotates, can fracture the femoral shaft.

With rare exceptions treatment should be conservative. A well-padded splint may be enough. If a circular cast is used it should be split, allowing the skin to be inspected daily for signs of pressure. Insufficient padding or failure to split a cast on a paralysed limb carries a high risk of producing pressure sores and painless ischaemia secondary to swelling. Immobilisation should not be prolonged as it is important to avoid joint stiffness, which might limit the patient's independence. It is particularly important to maintain the range of hip and knee movements, so that the patient's posture in the wheelchair is unaffected. Fortunately, fracture healing is usually satisfactory and callus formation good. There may, however, be an exacerbation of spasticity in the injured limb, which can complicate management of the fracture.

Post-traumatic syringomyelia (syrinx, cystic myelopathy)

Post-traumatic syringomyelia, an ascending myelopathy due to secondary cavitation in the spinal cord, is seen in at least 4% of patients. Symptoms may appear as early as two months after injury or in rare instances be delayed for over 30 years, the average latent period having previously been reported as eight to nine years.

The commonest presenting symptom is pain in the arm, usually unilateral, described as a dull ache but occasionally as burning or stabbing. The syrinx also often extends below the level of the spinal cord lesion, and in these instances bladder and bowel function can be further affected. The earliest sign is usually a dissociated sensory loss, with impaired or absent pain and temperature sensation (spinothalamic loss) and preservation of light touch and joint position sense (posterior column sparing). Some patients also have sensory loss over the face due to an extension of the cavitation into the upper cervical cord, which affects the spinal tract of the trigeminal nerve and, in rare instances, the brain stem. When present, motor loss is of a lower motor neurone type and is usually unilateral. Though there may be remissions, the condition may progress, perhaps even to the extent of converting low paraplegia into tetraplegia.

Though essentially clinical, the diagnosis is confirmed by magnetic resonance imaging (MRI) or in rare instances myelography with computed tomography (CT). Surgical treatment includes decompression or drainage of the syringomyelic cavity. Pain is usually relieved, but relief of sensory symptoms and motor loss is less predictable.

Pain

Pain relief in the acute stage of spinal cord injury has been discussed in chapters 1 and 4.

Chronic intractable pain after spinal cord injury is a particularly difficult problem, largely because of the profound emotional effect of a severe disability occurring suddenly and unexpectedly in a previously healthy and often young patient. A self-generating mechanism has been suggested for pain in the central nervous system, and it is possible, particularly in

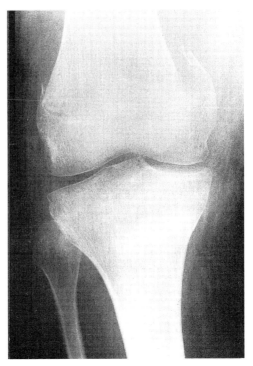

Figure 13.2 Supracondylar fracture of the right femur, the result of a "minor" fall in a patient with mid-thoracic paraplegia.

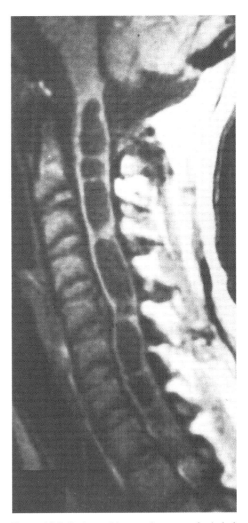

Figure 13.3 Patient with complete tetraplegia below C5 after fracture of C5 four years previously. She experienced further loss of function in the left arm. MRI showed extensive multilocular syrinx above and below the site of fracture.

patients with incomplete spinal cord lesions, that abnormal sensations arising adjacent to the site of cord damage will act as stimuli for the subsequent development of chronic pain. The "conditioning" effect of early acute pain on the nervous system can be minimised by a sympathetic attitude towards the patient and prompt administration of adequate doses of analgesics to relieve pain from the site of bony injury. The spine should be realigned, nerve root compression relieved if necessary, and the limbs correctly positioned and regularly put through a full range of passive movements.

During the first few weeks or months after injury discomfort or pain may occur, which appears to be related to neural damage rather than the musculoskeletal trauma. It may take one of several forms. There may be an unpleasant or painful sensation in a paralysed area similar to the phantom phenomenon experienced after amputation. Another example is an acute burning or stabbing sensation felt immediately below the neurological level of the lesion or several segments distally, which can be continuous and extremely incapacitating. This type of pain is often seen in cauda equina lesions. In incomplete lesions pain can also present as a burning sensation associated with hyperalgesia and may be increased by peripheral stimulation or movement of the limb. Pain that follows an anatomical distribution at or just below the level of the cord lesion may be due to damage at the root entry zone, but in these circumstances it is important to exclude nerve root compression, which may rarely require surgical decompression.

The number of patients who complain of severe chronic pain is considerable, and many others are aware of abnormal sensation below the level of the lesion. Continuing spinal instability must be treated, but otherwise mobilisation should begin as early as possible after injury, the distraction of full participation in a busy rehabilitation programme being the most helpful measure.

Most analgesics do not satisfactorily relieve pain associated with neural damage, although tramadol does appear to be of benefit in some patients. Tricyclic antidepressants combined with anticonvulsants, for example gabapentin or carbamazepine, often help. Treatment of sleep disturbance is important. Following psychological assessment and support, other techniques including transcutaneous nerve stimulation, acupuncture, relaxation techniques, and hypnotherapy can also be used. Spinal cord (dorsal column) stimulation appears to have little place in treatment. The effect of surgical techniques such as posterior rhizotomy and spinothalamic tractotomy, which interrupt the pain pathways, may only have a short lasting effect, and also have little place in treatment, but dorsal root entry zone coagulation (DREZ lesion) appears to be of benefit in selected patients. Surgery for pain management should be limited to a few specialist centres.

Sexual function

Sexual function depends on the level and completeness of the spinal cord lesion. If the lesion is incomplete sexual function may be affected to a varying degree and sometimes not at all. In women, although there is often an initial period of amenorrhoea after spinal cord injury, fertility is unimpaired. In men with complete or substantial spinal cord lesions, the ability to achieve normal erections, ejaculate, and father children can be greatly disturbed.

Erections

Most patients with complete upper motor neurone lesions of the cord have reflex, but not psychogenic, erections. However,

---

Box 13.4 Factors contributing to chronic pain

- Inadequate early pain relief of the spinal injury
- Spinal malalignment
- Nerve root compression
- Incompleteness of spinal cord lesion
- Poor emotional adjustment

Table 13.1 Proposed classification of pain related to spinal cord injury

Broad type (Tier 1)	Broad system (Tier 2)	Specific structures/pathology (Tier 3)
Nociceptive	Musculoskeletal	Bone, joint, muscle trauma or inflammation
		Mechanical instability
		Muscle spasm
		Secondary overuse syndromes
	Visceral	Renal calculus, bowel, sphincter dysfunction, etc.
		Dysreflexic headache
Neuropathic	Above level	Compressive mononeuropathies
		Complex regional pain syndromes
	At level	Nerve root compression
		Syringomyelia
		Spinal cord trauma/ischemia (segmental deafferentation, transitional zone, border zone, girdle zone etc.)
		Dual level cord and root trauma (double lesion syndrome)
	Below level	Spinal cord trauma/ischemia (central dysesthesia syndrome, central pain, phantom pain, etc.)

Reproduced with permission from Siddall PJ, Yezierski RP, Loeser JD. Pain following spinal cord injury: clinical features, prevalence and taxonomy. *International Assoc Study Pain Newsletter* 2000;3:3–7.

Box 13.5 Treatment of chronic pain

- Treat spinal instability and nerve root compression
- Distraction by busy rehabilitation programme
- Psychological support
- Antidepressants—for example, amitryptyline
- Anticonvulsants—for example gabapentin, carbamazepine
- Transcutaneous nerve stimulation
- Acupuncture
- Hypnotherapy and relaxation techniques
- Dorsal root entry zone coagulation (DREZ lesion)

Box 13.6 Spinal cord centres for sexual function

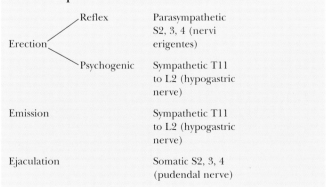

Erection	Reflex	Parasympathetic S2, 3, 4 (nervi erigentes)
	Psychogenic	Sympathetic T11 to L2 (hypogastric nerve)
Emission		Sympathetic T11 to L2 (hypogastric nerve)
Ejaculation		Somatic S2, 3, 4 (pudendal nerve)

the erections are not always sustained or strong enough for penetrative sex. In patients with complete lower motor neurone lesions parasympathetic connections from the S2 to S4 segments of the cord to the corpora cavernosa are interrupted, so that reflex erections are usually impossible.

Difficulty in achieving a satisfactory erection has been revolutionised by the introduction of sildenafil, which has often replaced the use of intracavernosal drugs such as alprostadil or vacuum erection aids and compressive retainer rings. Insertion of a penile implant is also possible, but carries a small risk of infection or erosion of the implant which will necessitate its removal. Some men with a sacral anterior nerve root stimulator are able to achieve stimulator-driven erections, in addition to using the stimulator primarily for micturition.

Emission and ejaculation

For seminal emission to occur the sympathetic outflow from T11 to L2 segments of the cord to the vasa deferentia, seminal vesicles, and prostate must be intact. Emission infers a trickling leakage of semen, with no rhythmic contractions of the pelvic floor muscles as in true ejaculation. Some patients with complete cord lesions at lumbar or sacral level may have both psychogenic erections and emissions.

If ejaculation is not possible during penetrative sexual intercourse, it may be induced by direct stimulation of the fraenum of the penis by masturbation or by using a vibrator. If this is unsuccessful, rectal electroejaculation may produce what is actually an emission.

In men who cannot ejaculate using the vibrator, or where electroejaculation is difficult, a hypogastric plexus stimulator can be implanted to obtain seminal emission, using a single inductive link across the skin. Men with lesions above T6 are at risk of autonomic dysreflexia developing during ejaculation. If this occurs activity should be curtailed, the man sat upright, and if necessary given sublingual nifedipine. Glyceryl trinitrate is also an effective treatment, but it is essential that patients are warned of the potentially fatal interaction of nitrates with sildenafil.

For men when neither emission nor ejaculation can be achieved it may be possible to collect spermatozoa by the technique of epididymal aspiration or testicular biopsy.

Preparation for sexual intercourse

Preparation for sexual intercourse includes ensuring that the bladder is as empty as possible. A man with an indwelling catheter should preferably remove it, but it may be strapped back on to the shaft of the penis. In the woman a catheter may be left in situ. The able-bodied partner tends to be the more active, and this has a bearing on the positions used for intercourse.

Fertility

Fertility is generally reduced in men after spinal cord injury. The sperm count is usually low, with diminished motility due to various factors, probably including continuing non-ejaculation, raised testicular temperature, and infection. The quality of the seminal fluid may improve with repeated ejaculations, however, and successful insemination has been reported both with the vibrator and by electroejaculation. It is essential to obtain microbiological cultures of the seminal fluid and to eradicate

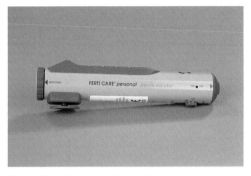

Figure 13.4 Ferticare vibrator for inducing seminal emission by penile stimulation.

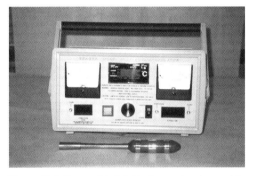

Figure 13.5 Seager Model 14 electroejaculator with rectal probe. By courtesy of Professor SWJ Seager, Washington DC, USA.

Box 13.7 Aids to sexual function and fulfilment in relationships

To enhance sexual expression:
- Use imagination, time and effort in touching parts of the body not affected by the injury, exploring both partners' preferences, experimenting with other erotic stimuli, etc.

For erection:
- Oral sildenafil
- Intracavernosal drugs
- Vacuum erection aid and compressive retainer ring
- Penile implant (small risk of infection or extrusion)
- Sacral anterior root stimulator

For ejaculation or seminal emission:
- Vibrator
- Electroejaculation unit
- Hypogastric plexus stimulator

To collect spermatozoa:
- Initial sperm culture
- Retrieve collected spermatozoa by epididymal aspiration

Further assisted conception techniques:
- Seminal fluid enhancement
- Intrauterine insemination
- *In vitro* fertilisation
- Intracytoplasmic sperm injection

To counteract autonomic dysreflexia:
(possible in men during ejaculation, and in women during labour, if lesion above T6)
- Sublingual nifedipine *or*
- Glyceryl trinitrate (potentially fatal interaction with sildenafil)

any infection prior to proceeding with any attempt at fertilisation. The success rate has recently improved with the use of assisted conception techniques, including enhancement of seminal fluid, intrauterine insemination, and assisted reproductive technology, such as *in vitro* fertilisation (IVF) and intracytoplasmic sperm injection (ICSI).

Labour

If the spinal cord lesion is complete above T10, labour may be painless and forceps delivery required because of inability to bear down effectively during the second stage of labour. Autonomic dysreflexia during labour is a risk in patients with lesions at T6 and above, but this complication can be prevented by epidural anaesthesia.

Fulfilment in relationships

It should be emphasised that emotional and psychological factors are as important as physical factors in a satisfying relationship and that such a relationship is possible even after severe spinal cord injury. This needs reiterating, particularly to young men who are otherwise apt to see their altered sexual function as a profound loss. Although sensation in the sexual organs may be reduced or absent, imaginative use can be made of touching and caressing, as areas of the body above the level of the spinal cord lesion may develop heightened sensation as erogenous zones. Some couples find that the extra time and effort required for sexual expression after one of them has suffered a spinal cord injury enriches their lives and results in a more understanding and caring relationship.

Further reading

- Biyani A, el Masry WS. Post-traumatic syringomyelia: a review of the literature. *Paraplegia* 1994;**32**:723–31
- Brinsden PR, Avery SM, Marcus S, Macnamee MC. Transrectal electroejaculation combined with *in-vitro* fertilization: effective treatment of anejaculatory infertility due to spinal cord injury. *Human Reproduction* 1997;**12**:2687–92
- Cross LL, Meythaler JM, Tuel SM, Cross AL. Pregnancy, labor and delivery post spinal cord injury. *Paraplegia* 1992;**30**:890–902
- Siddall PJ, Loeser JD. Pain following spinal cord injury. *Spinal Cord* 2001;**39**:63–73
- Tromans AM, Cole J. Sexual problems associated with spinal cord disease. In: Engler GL, Cole J, Merton WL, eds. *Spinal cord disease—diagnosis and management*. New York: Marcel Dekker, 1998, chap 28

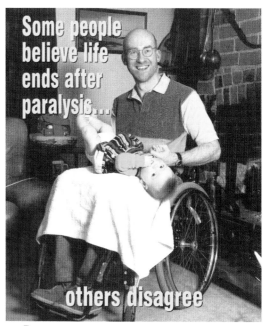

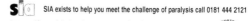

Figure 13.6 Produced with permission from Spinal Injuries Association.

14   Later management and complications—II

David Grundy, Anthony Tromans, John Hobby, Nigel North, Ian Swain

Later respiratory management of high tetraplegia

As a result of improved first aid at the scenes of accidents an increasing number of patients are surviving with neurological lesions above C4, who have therefore lost diaphragmatic function and can no longer breathe. These patients require long-term ventilatory support. Modern portable ventilators that use a 12-volt battery can be mounted on a wheelchair, allowing the patient a degree of freedom and independence. Speech is possible with an uncuffed tracheostomy tube around which air can escape to the larynx.

In a small number of these patients the anterior horn cells of the phrenic nerve are spared and it may be possible to implant a phrenic nerve stimulator to achieve ventilation. The advantages of electrophrenic respiration are that it is more physiological than positive pressure ventilation and it gives the patient more freedom, the equipment being much lighter than a mechanical ventilator. The disadvantages are that stimulation often cannot be sustained for 24 hours, a rest period overnight is necessary on a mechanical ventilator, and the implant is expensive. The long-term ventilator-dependent patient needs 24-hour care by a team of carers competent to undertake endotracheal suction, but not necessarily including a qualified nurse.

Psychological factors

In the acute stage of spinal cord injury an individual may experience a range of emotions such as numbness, despair, fear, hope, and anger. This emotional turmoil is often chaotic and disorganised. It may be further complicated by the enforced period of bed rest during which a state of sensory deprivation ensues. Following this early period anxiety and depression may become apparent in approximately one third of individuals. The frustrations associated with the physical limitations of such a severe injury are compounded by the fact that most patients are young and before injury led active lives, often expressing themselves mainly through physical activities. The sudden inability to continue in this manner and the need to lead a more ordered life can mean a very difficult and prolonged period of adjustment. Failure to recognise that this process can continue for as long as two or three years may damage the process of rehabilitation and the patient's ultimate resettlement. The patient needs time to come to terms with his or her new status and to make decisions about the future without undue pressure.

Detection of these psychological problems is vital in order to make appropriate referral. Psychological support and therapy has been shown to be very effective in improving mood and also later adjustment in individuals with spinal cord injury. Other psychological problems that may be present following injury include post-traumatic stress disorder in which an individual continually relives their accident and marked problems with memory, concentration, and problem solving.

Detection of these problems and the provision of psychological therapy will enable an individual to overcome

---

Box 14.1 High tetraplegia

- Improved first aid has increased number of high tetraplegics surviving scene of accident
- If lesion above C4, diaphragmatic function lost

Box 14.2 Chronic ventilation

- Electrophrenic respiration (diaphragmatic pacing)
- Mechanical "domiciliary" ventilation

Advantages of electrophrenic respiration
- More physiological than positive pressure ventilation
- More portable than positive pressure ventilation

Drawbacks of electrophrenic respiration
- Often stimulation cannot be sustained, necessitating rest period overnight on mechanical ventilator
- More expensive

Box 14.3 Psychological factors

Acute stage:
- Initial stress reaction
- Sensory deprivation

Later stages:
- Anxiety and depression
- Post-traumatic stress disorder
- Cognitive problems
- Detecting psychological problems
- Appropriate referral
- Family
- Psychological support and therapy

them, as well as improving the process of rehabilitation. The family of the patient may also experience psychological difficulties and as a result benefit from support and intervention. A holistic approach including a psychological perspective will not only benefit the patient and their family but will improve rehabilitation and ultimately the long-term emotional outcome of those individuals who sustain this type of injury.

The hand in tetraplegia

Most tetraplegic patients give priority to restoring hand function. Much can be done to improve function in these patients with tendon transfer surgery and functional electrical stimulation. Patients should be at least 12 months post-injury and have been neurologically stable for 6 months prior to surgical intervention. They should be in good general health and marked spasticity is a relative contraindication to surgery. Fixed hand contractures are also a contraindication as they will compromise the quality of result. Soft, mobile hands with a full passive range of motion in the joints are ideal.

The presence of sensation is important for the functional result and determines whether bi-manual tasks can be done easily. In the absence of sensation, vision replaces sensation: the patient can only concentrate on one hand at a time.

Two-thirds of tetraplegic patients are unable to extend their elbows. Restoration of elbow extension enables the patient to reach overhead and also facilitates wheelchair skills, for pressure relief and transfers. The posterior third of the deltoid muscle is usually used and its tendon is connected to the triceps tendon at the elbow. The result depends on the initial strength of the deltoid muscle.

Wrist extension is a vital prerequisite to hand (palmar) grasp and lateral pinch (key grip).

In C5 or high C6 patients, lateral pinch or key grip, as described by Moberg, is possible during wrist extension by tenodesing the flexor pollicis longus to the lower end of the radius and stabilising the interphalangeal joint. Wrist extension is achieved by transferring brachioradialis into carpi extensor radialis brevis. With the wrist extended the thumb will oppose the radial side of the index finger.

In lower C6 lesions or better, functional hand grasp may be restored with a passive flexor tenodesis. Active wrist extension is achieved, by transferring the brachioradialis into the insertion of extensor carpi radialis brevis. If wrist extension is active and the extensor carpi radialis longus and brevis are normally innervated, extensor carpi radialis longus may be transferred into the flexor digitorum profundus to achieve finger flexion. Brachioradialis may be transferred into flexor pollicis longus for thumb flexion.

Further surgical procedures include implantation of the NeuroControl Freehand system (see below), which is an upper limb neuroprosthesis suitable for C5 and upper C6 spinal cord injured patients, and procedures to achieve an intrinsic balance and improve hand function in lower cervical injuries.

Functional electrical stimulation

Following spinal cord injury, lower motor neurone pathways may remain intact and have the potential to be electrically stimulated. Functional electrical stimulation (FES) of paralysed muscles to restore function is becoming more commonly used, although only a few systems are commercially available, such as the NeuroControl Freehand system, the Handmaster, and the

Box 14.4 Good psychological support improves:

- Adjustment to injury
- Process of rehabilitation
- Long-term outcome

Box 14.5 Aims

To restore:
- Active elbow extension
- Wrist extension
- Hand opening
- Hand grasp
  Palmar grasp
  Lateral pinch
- Improved ability to perform acts of daily living

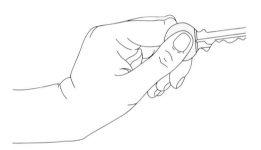

Figure 14.1 Key grip (lateral pinch).

Box 14.6 Factors in selection for surgery

Absolute prerequisites:
- Neurological level C5 and below
- No change in muscle power for at least 6 months
- Well motivated patient

Relative factors in selection:
- Adequate sensation in hand
- Minimal or no spasticity
- Minimal or no contractures

ODFS. The NeuroControl Freehand system consists of an implantable receiver placed subcutaneously on the pectoralis major fascia. Eight electrodes are attached to specific muscles to achieve hand opening, lateral pinch, and hand grasp. The implant is controlled by moving the opposite shoulder, which is connected by a lever to a "joystick" located on the central chest. These movements generate signals, which are analysed by a control unit which then provides output signals to the externally placed radiofrequency coil, thereby initiating hand opening and closing and grasp patterns. Functional grasp patterns improve the user ability to perform specific activities of daily living.

The Handmaster is a splint-based FES device for C5 tetraplegics. The forearm and wrist are held in a neutral position by the splint, on the inner surface of which are saline-soaked electrodes. These are placed over finger and thumb extensors and a thumb abductor, using pre-set patterns of stimulation to open and close the hand. The system is designed for holding objects such as a fork or pen.

Box 14.7 Functional electrical stimulation

Attempts to replace or improve missing functions, using the body's own muscles, through:
- External devices
- Implanted systems

Table 14.1 The practical uses of electrical stimulation to achieve function (FES)

Patient group	Stimulated function	Stimulator type	Control mechanism
Neurologically incomplete	Control of foot drop +\− knee extension, hip extension	ODFS (Odstock Dropped Foot Stimulator), with 1 or 2 channel external electrodes	Controlled by foot switch
	Respiration (there are three systems commercially available)	Implanted electrodes onto phrenic nerves	Pre-programmed
Neurologically complete	Bladder (bowel and erection)	NeuroControl Vocare bladder system (sacral anterior root stimulator—SARS)—implanted electrodes onto 2nd, 3rd and 4th anterior sacral nerve roots	Pre-programmed (3 options)
	Ejaculation	Implanted electrodes onto hypogastric plexus on sacrum	Pre-programmed
	Hand function (palmar and lateral grip, grasp and release)	Handmaster external system with surface electrodes	Pre-programmed triggered by pressing button
		NeuroControl Freehand implanted system with 8 electrodes on muscles of forearm and hand	Joystick attached to contralateral shoulder
		Research	
	Lower limbs (used for lower limb exercise, blood flow, skin quality, bone density and research into ambulation)	Surface electrodes	External feed back control system
		Implanted anterior lumbar and sacral nerve roots	External multi-option pre-programmed controller
		Implanted electrodes on muscle surface	External controller

NeuroControl Freehand and Vocare systems available from NeuroControl Corporation, 8333 Rockside Road, Valley View, Ohio 44125, USA. Tel: 00 1 216 912 0101.
Handmaster available from NESS (Neuromuscular Electrical Stimulation Systems Ltd), 19 Ha-Haroshet Street, PO Box 2500, Ra'anana 43654, Israel. Tel: 00972 9748 5738. Email: clinic@ness.co.il.
ODFS available from Department of Medical Physics and Biomedical Engineering, Salisbury District Hospital, Salisbury, Wiltshire SP2 8BJ, UK Tel: 01722 429065.

The Odstock Dropped Foot Stimulator (ODFS) is a single channel stimulator designed to correct dropped foot following incomplete spinal cord injury. Self-adhesive electrodes are placed over the common peroneal nerve as it passes over the head of the fibula. Stimulation is timed to the gait cycle using a pressure switch placed in the shoe. Trials of the ODFS have shown that walking can be less effort, faster, and safer.

The benefits of FES include an increase in muscle bulk and blood flow in the legs. This may be at the expense of spasms becoming stronger as muscular strength increases, but the majority of people find that their spasms are more predictable and less frequent, especially in the period immediately after FES.

Re-training muscles calls for a long-term commitment, and places great demands on the patient's time. Ambulation remains a distant goal for people with complete injuries, although cycling on recumbent tricycles is feasible. Systems in incomplete injuries can significantly improve walking speed and performance.

Ageing with spinal cord injury

The spinal cord injury population is ageing, partly because survival rates following injury have improved, and partly because the percentage of older people sustaining spinal cord injury has increased. The ageing spinal cord injured patient may present with several problems. In the case of people injured at a young age, if their parents are the carers, they will eventually be unable to cope, and may need care themselves.

The majority of patients will put increased strain on their upper limbs due to propelling their wheelchair, transferring or walking with crutches and orthoses, and often after 15–20 years will have increasing pain and discomfort in the joints of the upper limb, particularly the shoulders. They may then become less independent and have to consider using additional aids such as transfer boards, hoists, and mechanical aids to lift their chairs into their car. They may have to change from a manual to a motorised wheelchair, and have a vehicle which they can drive from their wheelchair. A change in lifestyle to reduce the number of transfers, further domestic modifications, and an increased level of care may be necessary. For those in employment, a reduction in the number of hours worked or the taking of early retirement may be inevitable. A person who has previously coped well with a severe disability for most of their life may begin to have very significant problems because of the effect of ageing.

Prognosis

It is important to indicate the probable degree of recovery at an early stage to both patient and relatives to make planning for the future realistic. The question of financial compensation will often arise in accident cases, and an informed opinion will be required on the degree of functional recovery that is likely and the effect on life expectancy. Recovery after a complete cord lesion is far less likely than after an incomplete lesion, but it is unwise to predict non-recovery too early, as some patients with an incomplete injury may initially appear to be totally paralysed because of spinal cord oedema and contusion, which later resolves. Forecasting the outcome in patients with an incomplete lesion is notoriously difficult. Too optimistic a prognosis may lead to great disappointment, with loss of morale and decreased interest in rehabilitation when hopes are unfulfilled. Contrary to a widely held view, however, neurological improvement can very occasionally be seen later

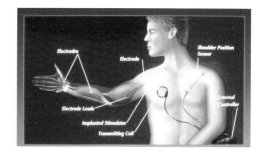

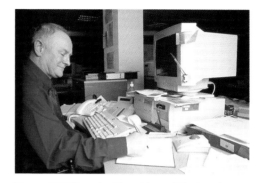

Figure 14.2 Top: the NeuroControl Freehand system. Bottom: a C6 tetraplegic patient at work using the Freehand system.

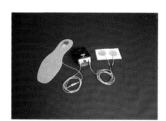
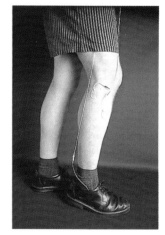

Figure 14.3 Left: the Odstock Dropped Foot Stimulator. Right: patient with incomplete spinal cord injury using the dropped foot stimulator.

Box 14.8 Neurological recovery

• Much less likely after complete lesion
• In incomplete lesions recovery may occur for two years or more

Table 14.2 Life expectancy in years for people with spinal cord injuries who survive at least one year after injury, according to current age and neurological category (Frankel grades—see box below)

Current age (years)	Normal*	C1–C4 (Frankel grade A, B, C)	C5–C8 (Frankel grade A, B, C)	T1–S5 (Frankel grade A, B, C)	(Frankel grade D)
5	70.8	45.0	52.0	59.5	63.0
10	65.9	40.5	47.3	53.7	58.2
15	61.0	36.1	42.6	49.0	53.4
20	56.3	32.8	38.6	44.8	49.0
25	51.6	29.9	34.7	40.8	44.7
30	46.9	26.8	30.7	36.7	40.5
35	42.2	23.7	27.0	32.7	36.1
40	37.6	20.9	23.6	28.8	31.7
45	33.0	18.4	20.4	25.1	27.5
50	28.6	15.5	17.0	21.2	23.4
55	24.4	12.8	13.8	17.3	19.5
60	20.5	11.0	11.2	13.8	15.9
65	16.9	8.8	8.8	10.9	13.2
70	13.6	6.6	6.6	8.3	10.4
75	10.7	4.7	4.7	6.1	8.0
80	8.1	3.1	3.1	4.2	6.1

*Normal values are from 1988 United States life tables for the general population.
Taken from DeVivo MJ, Stover SL, Long-term survival and causes of death.
In: Stover SL, *et al.* eds., *Spinal cord injury. Clinical outcomes from the model systems.* Gaithersburg: Aspen Publishers, 1995.

than two years after injury, not only with nerve root and cauda equina lesions but also with cord injuries.

Mortality in acutely injured patients managed in a spinal injuries unit is now less than 5%. Death within the first few days is likely to be from respiratory failure, particularly in high tetraplegia. The presence of multiple injuries, age, and previous health of the patient all play a part. In patients surviving the period immediately after injury pulmonary embolism is still the commonest cause of death in the acute phase.

With the modern management of spinal cord injury, particularly improvements in the management of the urinary tract and pressure sore prevention, life expectancy has improved over recent years; as a consequence pathologies experienced by the general population such as atherosclerosis and its complications, and malignancy, are now major causes of late death, as well as respiratory causes, particularly in tetraplegic patients.

Great progress has been made in the care of patients with spinal cord injuries since the 1940s, when spinal injuries units were first established. There has been a remarkable decrease in complications by using the multidisciplinary approach provided by such units, yet some patients are still denied referral. Unless complete recovery occurs, patients should have lifelong hospital outpatient follow up but with emphasis on continuing care and support in the community.

Although it is right to be optimistic about the future of these patients, their injuries can make a devastating change to their lives. In many cases the injuries need not have happened. For example, a high proportion of road traffic accidents is caused by alcohol consumption, high speeds, and dangerous driving, motorcyclists being particularly vulnerable. Ignorance of the danger of diving into shallow water results in many injuries to the cervical spine. Failure to take simple precautions in the home, such as ensuring that stairs are adequately lit at night for the elderly, may result in falls with cervical hyperextension injuries. Carelessness in contact sports can lead to serious injury. Recognition of this fact has led responsible authorities such as the Rugby Football Union to modify the laws of the game and issue advice on how it can be made safer, but

Box 14.9 Frankel grades

A "Complete"—total motor and sensory loss
B "Sensory only"—sensory sparing
C "Motor useless"—motor sparing of no functional value
D "Motor useful"—motor sparing of functional value
E "Recovery"—no functional deficit

From Frankel HL, Hancock DO, Hyslop G, *et al.* The value of postural reduction in the initial management of closed injuries of the spine with paraplegia and tetraplegia. *Paraplegia* 1969;**7**:179–92

Box 14.10 Many injuries are preventable

- Road traffic accidents associated with alcohol consumption and dangerous driving
- Diving into shallow water, resulting in tetraplegia
- Contact sports, e.g., rugby
- Some injuries are made worse by mishandling

much more could be done in other aspects of accident prevention, for instance in horse riding.

Finally, those who work with patients with spinal cord injuries are often impressed by the surprisingly high quality of life possible after injury. Many achieve a remarkable degree of independence, earn their own living, choose to marry, have children, and participate fully in family life. They may indeed have special qualities because they have successfully come to terms with their disability, and many will make a valuable contribution to society.

Further reading

- Brindley GS. The first 500 patients with sacral anterior root stimulator implants: general description. *Paraplegia* 1994;**32**:795–805
- Glass C. *Spinal cord injury: impact and coping.* Leicester: BPS Books, 1999
- North NT. The psychological effects of spinal cord injury: a review. *Spinal Cord* 1999;**37**:671–79
- Stover SL, DeLisa JA, Whiteneck GC, eds. *Spinal cord injury. Clinical outcomes from the model systems.* Gaithersburg: Aspen Publishers, 1995
- Whiteneck GC, Charlifue SW, Gerhart KA, Lammertse DP *et al.,* eds. *Aging with spinal cord injury.* New York: Demos, 1993
- Functional electrical stimulation: sources of information: <www.salisburyfes.com> FES clinical service and research at Salisbury District Hospital. Good links to other sites. <www.fes.cwru.edu> General FES information

15 Spinal cord injury in the developing world

Anba Soopramanien, David Grundy

Introduction

The situation in the developing world is characterised by a high incidence of spinal cord injuries and poor financial resources, which, in addition, may be unevenly distributed within countries and districts. Other health priorities make it difficult for decision makers to allocate significant means for spinal cord injury care and management. Staff are very often inadequately trained and have to work in a difficult environment with little financial reward. They often have to struggle in order to survive as individuals. Discharge planning can be difficult with lack of social help, poor housing conditions, and architectural and social barriers. Given all these challenges, how can we effectively care and provide for spinal cord injured patients in the Third World?

Incidence of spinal cord injury

The incidence of spinal cord injury is higher than in the western world. Factors that contribute to this include:

- poor road conditions
- poor servicing of vehicles
- high speed and unsafe driving
- lack of seat belts or headrests in cars
- corruption and bribery interfering with the implementation of traffic regulations
- overcrowded cars, shifting the centre of gravity of the cars
- abuse of alcohol and narcotic drugs
- widespread use of firearms in certain cultures
- inadequate safety measures when diving, playing contact sports, or repairing roofs
- unusual circumstances such as falling from a cart, from trees or accidents involving animals such as collisions with camels crossing the road.

It is, however, difficult to know the size of the problem given that proper epidemiological studies are lacking in most countries except the United States, where data has been relatively well collected. If the incidence can only be estimated in countries like France and the United Kingdom, it is no wonder that precise data is unavailable for developing countries. Rightly so, international funding agencies are not prepared to spend scarce resources in trying to obtain the exact figures when stress has to be laid on providing treatment.

There have been attempts in a few countries to portray a clearer picture of the situation. The available epidemiological studies have quoted the incidence for Russia, Romania, Turkey and Taiwan as 29.7, 30, 12.7 and 18.8 per million respectively. The incidence can vary within the same country as has been highlighted in a recent study on Turkey, and within different age groups. Thus in Taiwan with an annual incidence of 18.8 per million people, the incidence is 47.6 per million for the geriatric population.

These figures relate to the survival rate of those who sustain a spinal cord injury. An epidemiological study carried out in Portugal quotes the annual incidence as 57.8 new cases per million inhabitants, including those who died before being admitted to hospital, with an annual survival rate of 25.4 new

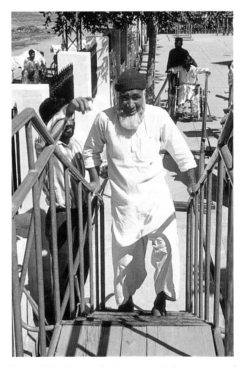

Figure 15.1 A paraplegic using training steps made of local material. From The International Committee of the Red Cross.

Box 15.1 The challenges

- Poor financial resources
- Other health priorities make it difficult to allocate significant means for spinal cord injury care
- Inadequately trained and poorly paid staff
- Inadequate social help
- Poor housing conditions
- Architectural and social barriers

Box 15.2 Incidence

- Epidemiological studies generally lacking
- Higher incidence than in western world
- Mostly paraplegic
- Predominantly young males

cases per million inhabitants. The death rate was very high during the first week, peaking during the first 24 hours. One would expect a higher global incidence of death for developing countries.

The causes of spinal cord injury vary from one country to another. Motor vehicle accidents accounted for 49% of spinal cord injuries in Nigeria, 48.8% in Turkey and 30% in the geriatric population in Taiwan. Falls from heights represented another major source of spinal cord injury with 36.5% in Turkey and 21.2% in Jordan. In Bangladesh the most common causes of traumatic lesions were falls while carrying a heavy weight on the head and road traffic accidents. Other causes included gunshot wounds (between 1.9% and 29.3% in Turkey), stab wounds (between 1.38% and 3.33% in Turkey, 25.8% in Jordan), and diving accidents.

In general 60% of patients were paraplegic and 40% tetraplegic. The mean age at injury was 30 years in Nigeria, 35.5 and 15.1 years in Turkey, 33 years in Jordan, and 10–14 years in Bangladesh. The male to female ratio was 10:1 in Nigeria, 1.7:1 in Taiwan, and 5.8:1 in Jordan. This points to a predominantly young male population being affected. They often are the "breadwinners" and the already precarious financial situation of the family can be further compromised by the sudden disappearance of the main source of revenue and subsistence.

Financial considerations

The situation is characterised by 80% of the world population having access to only 20% of the world's financial resources. There are big demands on these resources. Health has to compete with other areas and within health there are so many other priorities, so that rehabilitation needs are not easily met.

The mid-1998 world population stood at 5901 million inhabitants with 4719 million (80%) living in less developed regions. Asia accounted for 61% (3585 million), Africa for 749 million, and Latin America and the Caribbean 504 million. These figures will be increased as projected in Table 15.1.

A more detailed analysis shows that eight out of the ten countries having more than 100 million inhabitants are from the less developed regions. They include China (1256 million), India (982 million), Indonesia, Brazil, Pakistan, Russian Federation, Bangladesh, and Nigeria. The United States and Japan also have more than 100 million inhabitants. These countries allocate resources to the health of their citizens, according to their means and priorities, as in Table 15.2.

These figures point to the gross inequality between countries, which is further compounded by the inequality within each country. Furthermore it is estimated that of the world's 6 billion people, 2.8 billion live on less than 2US$ per day and 1.2 billion on less than 1US$ per day. Financial resources are therefore very scarce and priorities focus on maternal and child health, investing in a strong primary healthcare system, HIV and AIDS, clean water, and sanitation. It is doubtful whether substantial resources will ever be made available for spinal cord injury care. The only way to ensure that a reasonable standard of care is offered world wide is to be innovative in devising a strategy that will require as little financial means as possible.

Manpower and staffing issues

Rehabilitation medicine is often not as highly regarded as other specialities such as orthopaedic surgery. It may therefore be easier to find orthopaedic surgeons able to fix the spine, whether or not it is indicated, rather than spinal cord injury

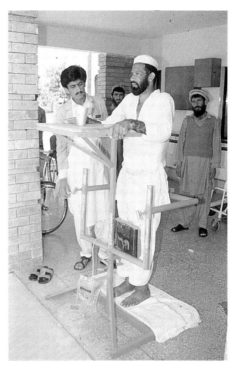

Figure 15.2 Standing frame made from metal rods available in the local market. From The International Committee of the Red Cross.

Table 15.1 Population ($\times 10^6$) of the major regions of the world. Source: UN Population Division: World Population Prospectus. The 1998 Revision

	1998	2050
World	5901	8909
More developed regions	1182	1155
Less developed regions	4719	7754
Africa	749	1766
Asia	3585	5268
Europe	729	628
Latin America/Caribbean	504	809
Northern America	305	392
Oceania	30	46

Table 15.2 Health expenditure per capita for selected countries. Source: World Health Report 2000, World Health Organisation, Geneva

Country	Health expenditure per capita in US dollars per year
United States of America	4187
Switzerland	3564
Germany	2713
France	2369
United Kingdom	1303
Brazil	319
Russian Federation	158
Nigeria	30
Indonesia	18
Pakistan	17
Bangladesh	13
Somalia	11

specialists. In many instances, surgery is isolated from rehabilitation, which might never be offered to the patient. Management of bladder, bowel and sexual function can be poorly organised, and skin care overlooked, leading to pressure sores. Patients can develop complications and die of chest or urinary infection or untreated autonomic dysfunction.

Nurses will be attracted to areas that are less physically demanding and labour intensive in countries where the use of hoists is not widespread and manual handling of patients is necessary. Physiotherapists are not always adequately trained, and can sometimes be physical training instructors who have only had a few months' training in the fundamentals of anatomy, physiology, and movement. Occupational therapy does not exist as a speciality in many countries. Social workers have little to offer in terms of state help. The other difficulties relate to a very low level of salaries, lack of equipment, and medication. This in turn may lead to demotivation and reinforce individualistic attitudes, whereas the focus should have been on teamwork.

Social, psychological and architectural barriers

Among the major obstacles to successful rehabilitation of spinal cord injury are social issues and the way society views disability. The social barriers include limited financial means available within the community, and the household not allowing survival with dignity; changing social roles when a "breadwinner" loses his job, physical independence and status within the family; stress on the family who have to find new human and other resources to look after the disabled; struggle with the physical environment within and around the house. In addition, wheelchairs may not be available, or are too expensive.

The way society views disability is a reflection of social and religious values. In certain cultures, disability is viewed as a punishment for past sins. In others, disabled people may not be allowed to enter certain religious sites if they are incontinent of urine or faeces and considered "unclean or soiled". Religious considerations may be so important that—for patients not to be excluded from their environment—they dictate how the paralysed bladder and/or bowel will be managed.

Prejudice is widespread against the disabled person, who is pitied. By acquiring a spinal cord injury, a person becomes part of a group he or she was previously looking down upon. Disabled people are at times hidden from mainstream life and cared for in a separate environment within the family dwelling. It is not common to see a disabled person going out shopping, to the cinema, or participating in active life. Little has been done to empower the individual or give him or her a voice. The tendency has been for charitable organisations to provide institutional help and care, thus appeasing social conscience, but not promoting dignity, individual expression, and choice. Some societies take pride in promoting the view that their system is acceptable, with the extended family taking up an active new, supportive role, but many problems exist "behind closed doors".

Substantial financial resources are not expected to become available; they may even become scarcer. Social and religious values are deep-rooted and might not be easy to change, and it would be unrealistic to believe that we can do much about changing the physical environment to bring it to the level of developed societies with wide pavements, roads, streets, slopes, doors, and rooms all wheelchair friendly.

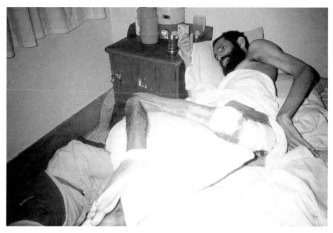

Figure 15.3 Emaciated patient with pressure sores and contractures. From The International Committee of the Red Cross.

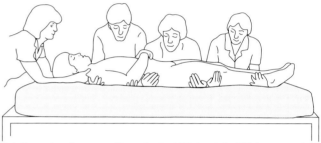

(a) Preparing for a coordinated spinal lift (straight lift) in a tetraplegic. The person holding the head and neck directs the procedure.

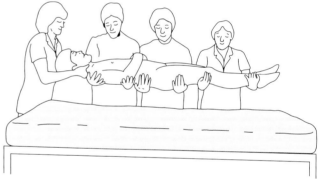

(b) Straight lift in a tetraplegic.

Figure 15.4 Manual handling.

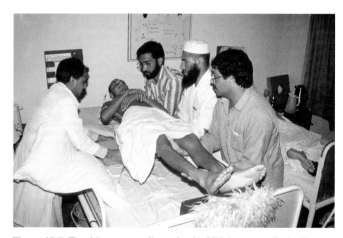

Figure 15.5 Teaching a co-ordinated spinal lift in a paraplegic. From The International Committee of the Red Cross.

Providing for the needs of spinal cord injured patients in developing countries

Any rehabilitation programme for spinal cord injured patients needs to address the issues highlighted above. We suggest a national strategy to look at and address the global picture, and local initiatives and implementation for increased efficiency and ownership. The international community has a duty and responsibility to provide help, expertise and support.

When planning the strategy, care must be taken not to blindly apply the methodology used in the developed world, but to adapt the principles of treatment to take into account the specificity of the Third World, especially the limited financial means and cultural differences. Much of what has been addressed in this book will be applicable to Third World countries: relevant topics will include clinical and neurological assessment; principles of management by nurses, physiotherapists and occupational therapists; bladder and bowel management; home adaptations. However, there will be no powered turning beds, and little or no physiotherapy and occupational therapy equipment. Handling of patients will be manual as in Figure 15.4. Surgical expertise and equipment as well as medication may be lacking. In some countries, enthusiasm to create sophisticated, well-equipped rehabilitation centres may be misplaced. It is essential to be innovative and use the principles of low-cost technology and self-reliance (principally on local, including human, resources). These principles have been successfully applied in two Red Cross projects: manufacturing wheelchairs, orthopaedic devices and therapy equipment using pipes, bicycle wheels and other local materials; using conservative management as often as possible to treat spinal fractures, particularly as surgery is so much more expensive and at times unnecessary; investing in training of staff and relatives/carers.

A comprehensive programme will focus on the following areas:

- Prevention of spinal injuries, using all available media and modes of communication.
- Education of the general public on suspecting spinal injuries at the sites of accidents, together with the development of means to improve handling, lifting and transportation of patients.
- Designation of a few hospitals to be the referral centres for the specialised treatment of spinal injuries.
- Training of staff within the hospitals and the community both in individual, professional skills and to work within a multidisciplinary team.
- Provision of the required specialist tools, using the principles of low-cost technology and self-reliance.
- Involvement of carers and relatives in managing patients in hospital, and training them in areas such as turning, positioning of patients, chest physiotherapy, and bladder and bowel evacuation.
- Setting up appliance services to manufacture at low cost: wheelchairs, orthoses such as cervical and thoracolumbar braces, and drop-foot devices.
- Offering psychological and social support to patients to deal with acute problems and those anticipated at their discharge. Incorporating psychological interventions to help individuals cope with their disability, and the community (key family members and religious or spiritual leaders) to be more aware of disability issues. Thus there could be a shift towards more empowerment of the disabled so that they can have a greater say in their destiny instead of being "assisted".

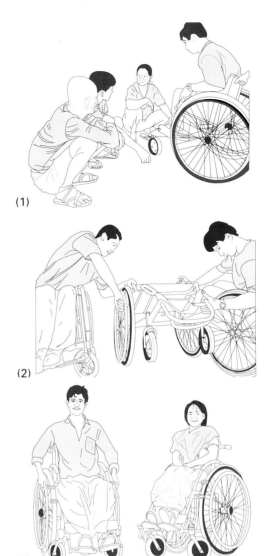

Figure 15.6 (1) "Mekong" Cambodia wooden wheelchair. (2) Teaching wheelchair assembly in Sri Lanka. (3) Two locally made wheelchairs, Bangladesh.

Box 15.3 Comprehensive programme

- Prevention of spinal injuries
- Education of general public
- Training of staff, carers, and relatives
- Use of principles of low-cost technology (using local materials when possible) and self-reliance
- Being innovative in overcoming discharge barriers

- Identification of discharge problems: architectural barriers within the house/flat and community, and means of overcoming them using all resources available nationally and locally.
- Organising access to medical help within the local community, and long-term follow-up of discharged patients.
- The international community with support from international organisations (World Health Organisation, United Nations, World Bank, Non-Governmental Organisations) will help in providing exchanges of ideas, experience, technical know-how, especially in the areas of appropriate technology, and training of hospital and community staff. Of relevance will be the organisation of regional seminars, and the publication of teaching materials.

Conclusions

It would be fair to acknowledge the hard work of a few individuals and non-governmental organisations in many parts of the world. Their contributions have undoubtedly impacted positively on the lives of a significant number of people with spinal cord injury. The world needs to learn from their experience. It is essential to devise a strategy that will allow access to care for spinal cord injury patients worldwide, bearing in mind the limited financial means and the social, psychological, architectural barriers that will not change significantly in years to come.

Useful addresses

Dr Anba Soopramanien, The Duke of Cornwall Spinal Treatment Centre, Salisbury District Hospital, Salisbury SP2 8BJ. Tel: 44 1722 429007; fax: 44 1722 336550; email: Dr.A.Soopramanien@shc-tr.swest.nhs.uk

Handicap International, 14 Av. Berthelot, 69361 Lyon Cedex 017, France. Tel: 00 33 478 697979; fax: 00 33 478 697994; email: programmes@handicap-international.org

International Committee of the Red Cross, Geneva, 19 Avenue de la Paix, CH 1202 Geneva, Switzerland. Tel: 41 22 7346001; fax: 41 22 7332057; email: review.gva@icrc.org

International Federation of the Red Cross, Geneva, PO Box 372, CH 1211 Geneva 19, Switzerland. Tel: 41 22 7304222; fax: 41 22 7330395; email: secretariat@ifrc.org

International Medical Society of Paraplegia, National Spinal Injuries Centre, Stoke Mandeville Hospital, Mandeville Road, Aylesbury, Bucks. Tel: 44 1296 315866; fax: 44 1296 315870; email: imsop@bucks.net; www.imsop.org.uk

Motivation (Wheelchair charity), Brockley Academy, Brockley Lane, Bakewell, Bristol BS19 3AQ. Tel: 44 1275 464017; fax: 44 1275 464019; email: motivation@motivation.org.uk

World Bank, 1818 H Street, N.W. Washington D.C. 20433, United States. Tel: 202 477 1234; fax: 202 477 6391; email: feedback@worldbank.org

World Health Organisation, 1211 Geneva 27, Switzerland. Tel: 4122 791 2111; fax: 41 22 791 4870; email: info@who.int

Further reading

- Chen H, Chen S-S, Chiu W-T *et al.* A nation-wide epidemiological study of spinal cord injury in geriatric patients in Taiwan. *Neuroepidemiology* 1997;**16**:241–7

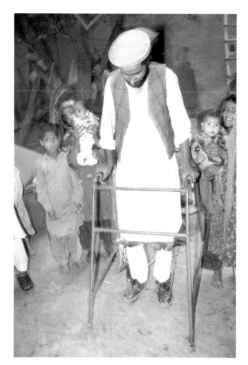

Figure 15.7 A walking frame made from water pipes. From The International Committee of the Red Cross.

- Hoque MF, Grangeon C, Reed K. Spinal cord lesions in Bangladesh: an epidemiological study 1994–1995. *Spinal Cord* 1999;**37**: 858–61
- Igun GO, Obekpa OP, Ugwu BT, Nwadiaro HC. Spinal injuries in the plateau state, Nigeria. *East Afr Med J* 1999;**76**:75–9
- Karacan I, Koyunku H, Pekel Ö *et al.* Traumatic spinal cord injuries in Turkey: a nation-wide epidemiological study. *Spinal Cord* 2000;**38**:697–701
- Karamechmetoglu S, Ünal S, Kavacan I *et al.* Traumatic spinal cord injuries in Istanbul, Turkey. An epidemiological study. *Paraplegia* 1995;**33**:469–71
- Martins F, Freitas F, Martins L *et al.* Spinal cord injuries—epidemiology in Portugal's Central Region. *Spinal Cord* 1998;**36**:574–8
- Otom AS, Doughan AM, Kawar JS, Hattar EZ. Traumatic spinal cord injuries in Jordan—an epidemiological study. *Spinal Cord* 1997;**35**:253–5
- Silverstein B, Rabinovich S. Epidemiology of spinal cord injuries in Novosibirsk, Russia. *Paraplegia* 1995;**33**:322–5
- Soopramanien A. Epidemiology of spinal injuries in Romania. *Paraplegia* 1994;**32**:715–22

Acknowledgements

We thank Richard Bolton and colleagues of the Department of Medical Photography, Salisbury District Hospital, Salisbury, UK and Louise Goossens of the Photographic Unit, Wellington School of Medicine and Health Sciences, Ofago University, New Zealand, for the photographs.

Index

Page numbers in **bold** refer to figures; those in *italic* refer to tables or boxed material

Index

Index

Index